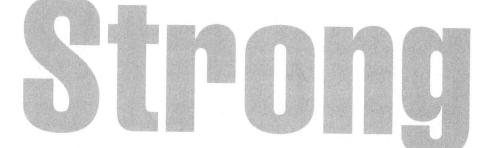

Strong

Nine Workout Programs for Women to Burn Fat, Boost Metabolism, and Build Strength for Life

Lou Schuler and
Alwyn Cosgrove

AVERY
AN IMPRINT OF PENGUIN RANDOM HOUSE
New York

AVERY

an imprint of Penguin Random House LLC
375 Hudson Street
New York, New York 10014

First trade paperback edition 2016
Copyright © 2015 by Lou Schuler and Alwyn Cosgrove
Photographs © 2015 by Michael Tedesco

Most Avery books are available at special quantity discounts for bulk purchase
for sales promotions, premiums, fund-raising, and educational needs.
Special books or book excerpts also can be created to fit specific needs.
For details, write SpecialMarkets@penguinrandomhouse.com.

The Library of Congress has catalogued the hardcover edition as follows:

Schuler, Lou.
Strong : nine workout programs for women to burn fat, boost metabolism, and build
strength for life / by Lou Schuler and Alwyn Cosgrove.
p.   cm.
ISBN 978-1-58333-575-8 (hardcover)
1. Exercise for women.   2. Weight training for women.   3. Women—Health and
hygiene.   I. Cosgrove, Alwyn.   II. Title.
RA781.S288   2015   2015015248
613.7'1082—dc23

ISBN 978-0-399-57343-9 (paperback)

Printed in the United States of America
1   3   5   7   9   10   8   6   4   2

BOOK DESIGN BY TANYA MAIBORODA

For my mom, Dorothy Schuler. Vice versa. (L.S.)
For Grandma Peggy, my greatest fan.
Thank you for always being on my team. (A.C.)

Contents

PART 1

WHAT WORKS, WHAT DOESN'T, AND WHY WE'RE STILL CONFUSED

PART 2

THE TRAINING PROGRAM

PART 3

THE EXERCISES

PART 4

YES, BUT . . .

Acknowledgments

ALTHOUGH THIS BOOK ISN'T A SEQUEL to *The New Rules of Lifting for Women*—we wrote it as a stand-alone training guide for women, including those who've never heard of us or seen our work—it wouldn't exist if not for the many readers who enthusiastically embraced that earlier book. Your continued support is beyond anything my coauthors and I anticipated, and I can never thank you enough.

Next I want to thank my coauthor, Alwyn Cosgrove, whose nine ass-kicking workout programs are the heart of this book, along with Megan Newman and Gigi Campo at Avery. My first phone conversation with Megan was in October 2004, and the fact that we're still working together eleven years later makes me the luckiest writer in my field. Photographer Michael Tedesco is another crucial member of our team. He and Matt Minor did an incredible amount of work in our two-day shoot, as did Jessi Kneeland, our strong, cheerful, and seemingly inexhaustible model. We wouldn't have had a place to shoot if not for the generosity of John Graham and his team at St. Luke's Sports and Human Performance Center in Allentown, including Brian Zarbatany, Jackie Bolig, Jeff Baker, Steve Hultgren, Jess Gaal, James Farley, and Lisa Cote. Thanks also to David Black and Sarah Smith at the David Black Agency; to Chris Turney and Geralyn Coopersmith at Nike; to Chris Poirier at Perform Better and Dave Barr at the NSCA; and to Gregg Stebben, whose promotion of the original *New Rules of Lifting* in 2006 gave us our first hint of the audience waiting for *NROL for Women*, which Gregg helped us launch so successfully two years later.

As always, I'm indebted to the many experts who help me understand research and practices that are far removed from my editorial training. At the top of the list are Stu Phillips, Bret Contreras, Bryan Chung, Dr. Spencer Nadolsky, Chad Waterbury, Mike T. Nelson, Greg Nuckols, Eric Cressey, Mike Roussell, Brad Schoenfeld, Alan Aragon, Susan Kleiner, and Nick Tumminello. Thanks also to Adam Campbell, Nick Bromberg, Sol Orwell, Dave Tropeano, Jon Goodman, Roland Denzel, and Kevin Larrabee; to Jeannine Trimboli, Dana Smith, Lisa Lilge, Brynda Ivan, and all the readers who've shared their stories with me over the years; to Cassandra Forsythe, our *NROL for Women* coauthor; and of course to my wife, Kimberly Heinrichs, and our three children.

L.S.

To the badass ladies of the NROL for Women Facebook groups: This one is for you.

Lou: I bet you never thought when you met me over lunch at a seminar twenty-odd years ago that we'd end up publishing six books together. You have no idea how much I appreciate your belief in me. Let's do six more.

Craig Rasmussen: Thanks for your help with these programs, for overseeing the program design at Results Fitness, and for writing my own programs. You took what started as my programming to a different level. You are, without a doubt, one of the greatest fitness professionals I've ever met, and the Results Fitness secret weapon.

Results Fitness: my team, my family, and my home. Thanks for being part of the journey.

Results Fitness University: the single greatest group of fitness professionals on the planet. Thank you for being part of our mission to change the way fitness is done.

To God, and in no small part Dr. Sven De Vos and the elite team of doctors and nurses at UCLA who saved my life and gave me these extra days here: I'll confess I don't know why I deserve these days, but I'll never take them for granted and will always treat them as a gift. We know for sure this book wouldn't exist if it weren't for you.

To Derek Campbell, my tae kwon do instructor and original mentor: You are the greatest human being I've ever met. You changed the direction of my life and remain my single biggest coaching influence. You took a kid with no future, taught him for free when his family had no money, and turned him into a champion. Just because you could. If I can ever be half the coach you are, I'll be ecstatic.

Team 164: I'll never forget where I came from. You have supported me from day one.

Terry: I hope I've never changed. Despite the fact we have been apart for years, every time we get together I feel like I saw you ten minutes ago.

Darren: I have no idea why we never got deported. You are a friend who knows all my darkest secrets (and, shockingly enough, are still my friend).

Robert: Am I the only one who calls you that? Thanks for teaching me so much and being in my corner for over a decade. And for making sure I don't miss a single funny thing ever posted on the Internet.

Rach: Still. Always. Forever. You're the best thing that's ever happened to this wee boy from Scotland. What a journey.

Mum: I wish you could see everything I've done. I really hope you can.

A.C.

Introduction: You Aren't Who You Used to Be

DANA SMITH REMEMBERS THE FIRST TIME. It was late summer 2009. "The arthritis in my knees was getting so bad my doctor was ready to put me on constant pain meds," she told me recently. "I told him I'd think about it and get back to him."

Thinking about it meant research. Research convinced her that it was time to take action. Specifically, to strengthen her muscles with a serious training program. That led her to *The New Rules of Lifting for Women*, a book my coauthors and I had published the year before. We wrote it for a simple reason: Readers asked us for it. They asked because the guidance women received from the media, from their peers, and even from fitness professionals in health clubs was the opposite of what we provided for men.

This was despite the fact there was no reason to give different advice to men and women. Exercise science had concluded long before that the muscles of men and women are exactly the same. Your muscles and my muscles perform the same actions and produce the same movements. Pound for pound, they generate the same amount of force. When trained, they respond equally well. But here's the worst part: This wasn't secret information. Everyone who wrote about strength training or trained female athletes or worked with female clients either knew or should have known.

The exercises in *NROL for Women* weren't the ones readers like Dana were used to seeing in books and magazines. She'd never done a push-up before, or a deadlift, or a squat with a barbell on her back. And the advice to focus on strength and muscle development, rather than "toning" and "shaping," was a paradigm shift for women who'd developed an irrational fear of "bulking up" if they lifted anything bigger than their forearms or heavier than a purse.

So on September 9, 2009, Dana tried it. Arthritic joints and all. She could barely bend her knees on the squat and had to do her push-ups against a kitchen counter. But by the end of the program, she could do eight push-ups. *Traditional* push-ups, with her hands and toes on the floor. She could lift a 135-pound barbell off the ground and squat with 100 pounds on her back. And those pain meds her doctor was about to prescribe? Turns out, she didn't need them. She just needed to get strong.

"Anyone who actually finishes the program comes out a changed person," she told me. "Most of us never knew how strong we could be. It opened doors we didn't even know were there."

OUR GREATEST MISTAKE

Here's the irony of Dana's transformation: We never thought readers like her would pick up the book. The original title, *Lift Like a Man, Look Like a Goddess*, signaled our goal of reaching women who were already working out but not getting the results they wanted. I saw countless women like that in the gym. They were healthy and appeared able and willing to work hard toward their goals, but did so with workouts that were unlikely to help them accomplish anything useful. Those are the readers who contacted Alwyn and me when we published *The New Rules of Lifting*, our first book together, in 2006.

To our delight, *NROL for Women* (the title we very wisely switched to after the book was already written and photographed) reached that target audience. We heard from readers who'd lost fat, improved their physiques in noticeable ways, and found they enjoyed doing the type of workouts we provided for guys in the original *NROL*.

But we also heard from readers like Dana, who was so excited by her progress that she started a Facebook group for her fellow lifters. Beyond their gender and the fact that they love lifting heavy things, they have little in common. In fact, these days I rarely hear from anyone who fits my original concept. Our universe of lifters includes women from their twenties to their seventies. From competitive athletes to complete beginners. From underweight to severely obese. From healthy to anything but.

You'd think it would be the ultimate ego trip for an author. Who doesn't want to see his book take on a life of its own, with readers he never thought would be interested in the topic he writes about? And on a good day, sure, it's flattering. More often, the readers I hear from remind me of all the things I could've done better. (I won't bother listing them here, but if you're curious, you can check out our online reviews.) The success of *NROL for Women* allowed us to expand the series to five books, each one reflecting the evolution of Alwyn's training strategy and workout design, developed with his wife, Rachel, and their staff at Results Fitness in Santa Clarita, California. When their philosophy shifted to include more mobility and core training, we wrote *NROL for Abs*. When readers asked us for programs targeted to older, heavier, or otherwise nontraditional lifters, we wrote *NROL for Life*. And then we put together Alwyn's entire system—including 10 total-body programs—for our fifth book, *Supercharged*.

With each book, the breadth of our readership expanded in every direction. We hear from beginners who have more challenges to overcome than typical newbies. We hear from serious athletes who need to get stronger for their sport. And more and more, we hear from readers of our previous books who ask the toughest question of all: "Now that I'm no longer what I used to be, what's my next step?"

Why is it so tough to answer? Because it's one Alwyn and I struggle with every single day.

THE PEOPLE WE USED TO BE

I've been writing about exercise, nutrition, and health since 1992, when I started at *Men's Fitness* magazine in Los Angeles. After six years at *MF* I moved across the country with my pregnant wife and two-year-old son to take a job at *Men's Health*. Six years (and two daughters) later, I went out on my own, writing the NROL series with Alwyn and contributing to a long list of magazines and websites.

Writing about strength training was a lucky break, a rare chance to merge my skills and interests. I started working out when I was 13, when I was usually the skinniest, weakest, and slowest kid who was actually interested in playing sports and chasing girls (most of whom could outrun me). I loved lifting almost from the start, but I was never especially good at it. Even at my strongest I was never actually *strong*. Not by meathead standards, anyway. In my youth I struggled to get bigger, and in middle age I fought to stay lean. Now, in my fifties, I see it as a war on three fronts, with body fat on the attack and strength and muscle mass in full retreat.

But that's nothing compared to what Alwyn has been through. Unlike me, Alwyn was an elite competitive athlete during his formative years in Scotland. He was a seven-time British champion in tae kwon do, and won two bronze medals as the UK's representative in the European championships. He moved to the United States, built a reputation as a personal trainer, and opened Results Fitness with Rachel. Then came cancer. Stage 4 lymphoma. He was told he was in remission after the first bout, but the cancer returned just 12 months later, right about the time we began work on *NROL for Women*. In real-estate terms, the stem-cell transplant that saved his life was a teardown. The procedure demolished his immune system, right down to the foundation, and then started over with healthy white blood cells.

That was in 2006, but he feels the effects to this day, and until recently he berated himself in almost every workout. "This is shit," he'd say after struggling through a set of squats or deadlifts. "When I was fighting, I wouldn't even warm up with this."

Then one day he had an epiphany. He told me about it when we got together to plan this book:

"If you ask a woman how much she weighs, you get a story, right? She'll tell you, 'When I was in high school, I weighed 135.' If you ask a guy how much he can deadlift, he'll tell you, 'When I was in college, I deadlifted 400.'"

In both situations, Alwyn would redirect the client: How much do you weigh *now*? How much can you deadlift *now*? So what would he say to a 41-year-old client who focused relentlessly on what he could do two decades, one continent, and two cancer diagnoses ago? He'd say something like this:

"Let's start over. Pretend you've never lifted before. Give yourself a clean scorecard. Every workout, every lift, is a new record. Five squats with good form? It's a new record. Well done. You got six on the next set? Same weight, same technique? Outstanding. That's another record, your second one today. Let's move on."

Moving on, in fact, is essential to your success in *Strong*.

If You're a Beginner . . .

You may already feel as if you're lost, like you jumped into the middle of someone else's conversation. Even if you're not a beginner, but this is your first structured training program, you may wonder if this is all going to be over your head. Trust me, it's not. Alwyn and I worked hard to make sure anyone can use his program, as long as you're willing to work hard and accept the fact that serious training requires a learning curve. You'll sometimes feel a little awkward as you learn new movements and get used to the equipment.

Appendix A, on p. 251, walks you through some of the basic terminology we'll use in *Strong*. (If you're reading this on a screen, you'll find the link in the Contents.) Appendix B, on p. 255, explains the equipment you'll need to do the workouts. And Appendix C, on p. 262, explains why there's never a good answer to one of the most frequently asked questions: How much weight should I use?

HOW TO USE THIS BOOK

Strong is divided into four sections:

Part One describes why it's so important to build strength and improve muscle quality, which means developing muscles that are bigger than they are now. I'll also look at weight management vs. weight loss, the importance of protein, and why so many of us (including some people who should know better) are still confused about health, fitness, and nutrition.

Part Two is Alwyn's new program, which I'll talk about in a moment.

Part Three describes and illustrates all the exercises you'll use, along with alternatives and options for many of them, concluding with a chapter on how (and whether) to incorporate other types of exercise.

Part Four attempts to anticipate your lingering questions.

Some of you will skip right over the opening chapters in Part One, and I promise I won't be offended. Those chapters, by necessity, include basic information about strength, muscle development, and weight control. But because the science of human performance continually expands, our understanding of the best way to apply it evolves. Over time, even the basics don't seem quite so basic anymore.

Speaking of science, the final section of the book, Notes, explains where I got the information I used in each chapter. So if you see a reference to "a recent study in the

Journal of Things You Try Not to Think About" or what "researchers at the University of Clickbait" discovered, and you'd like to know more, that's where you'll find it.

THE *STRONG* CHALLENGE

The core of this book is Alwyn's training program. The program has three phases. Each phase includes three stages. Each stage includes about a month's worth of workouts, if you do the recommended three workouts a week (each of which should take 50 to 60 minutes). On paper, that's nine months of training programs. But for most readers, it'll be at least a year's worth of actual training, which I'll explain in a moment. First, let's look at the three phases.

Phase One: Develop

In keeping with the theme of this introduction, Alwyn wants everyone to start with Phase One. For many of you, this goes without saying. But for the more experienced readers, especially veterans of one or more NROL programs, it doesn't make as much sense. If you aren't a beginner, why would you start at the beginning?

I answer this question in more detail in Chapters 6 and 7, but this is the short version: The more advanced you are, the more challenging the Phase One workouts will be. That's because you'll be able to use heavier weights and push yourself to a deeper level of fatigue. Remember, you're setting records each time.

If you *are* a beginner, don't be intimidated by phrases like *deeper level of fatigue* or all the talk about deadlifts and squats and other exercises you don't yet know how to do. You will. We're not throwing you into the deep end. You have plenty of time to get the hang of it.

As written, each stage in Phase One will take four weeks. (There's also a Special Workout in between Stage 1 and Stage 2, which you'll see in Chapter 7.) But it's okay to spend more time in each stage, especially if you're still getting stronger from one workout to the next. More advanced lifters, on the other hand, will adapt faster and will probably do better with just three weeks per stage.

Phase Two: Demand

Each of the three stages in Phase Two offers four weeks' worth of workouts that will be challenging to readers at all levels of experience. Alwyn describes them as "the badass stuff." For those who are new to the iron game, you'll improve your lifting skills while building strength and stamina. For those with more experience, you'll push yourselves with higher-volume workouts and techniques that challenge your perceived limits.

Phase Three: Display

Now, in Phase Three, you'll train for pure strength and performance. The goal is to establish new personal records (PRs). These benchmarks could be true PRs—that is, the most you've ever pressed, squatted, or deadlifted. Or they could be the best you can do now, at your current age and in your present circumstances. Whatever they are, they're real, and we hope you'll celebrate . . . for a week or two.

Then it's time to get back to work. Most readers should be able to repeat the program at least once, and get better results the second time through. Some of you may do even better the third time. Thus, for newer lifters, the *Strong* program can keep you busy for the foreseeable future.

HOW TO SUCCEED

Let's return to Dana Smith for a moment. In her years of moderating a lively Facebook group, she's noticed a trend: Those who follow Alwyn's *NROL for Women* program *as written* have the most success. Those who get frustrated and quit, she told me, have a common trait: They focus on the parts they don't like. They want to go back to whatever they were doing before, even if it wasn't working for them. I've noticed a parallel trend in some of the more critical feedback I receive: The readers who like the program the least try to modify it the most and achieve the fewest benefits.

This isn't to imply there's any such thing as a perfect program. Alwyn will be the first to tell you he's never written a program he didn't eventually figure out how to improve. But he'd also tell you this: Most of the time, you'll get better results if you commit to *any* program, however imperfect, and work your tail off on it, versus hopping from one system to the next in hopes of finding one that clicks. Persistence is what makes the magic happen.

But it's not really magic. It's just what you get when you push yourself from where you are now toward whatever your potential might be. That potential is a moving target through life. It's very different when you're young and unencumbered, and have the time and energy to train as long as you want and as hard as you want, compared to your potential after giving birth. Or when you have a demanding job. Or you're dealing with stressful life events or recovering from an injury, or when you're finally ready to describe yourself as middle-aged (which, trust me, is about the time others start to describe you as old).

That's why the best gift you can give yourself is a clean slate. Starting with the first workout of Phase One, every weight you lift on every exercise is a new personal record, because it's the most you can do *now*. No, you aren't who you used to be. But with time, effort, and the occasional callus on your palms, you'll ensure that who you are now is stronger than the person you were when you started the program.

PART 1

What Works, What Doesn't, and Why We're Still Confused

Why Strength Matters

For as long as I can remember, I wanted to be big and strong. And for good reason: Among men, there's a pecking order based on upper-body size. Men who appear more formidable are thought to be more dangerous, and the seemingly dangerous dude gets a lot of advantages. As a kid he's the first one picked in sports and the last one messed with by bullies. Men and women are more likely to see him as a leader. The bigger his upper body, the more romantic partners he'll have, and the earlier he'll start having them.

But for women, there's no such evolutionary logic behind the quest for strength. There are still plenty of health-related reasons to train for it. (I'll get to those in a moment.) But for most women, the decision to get stronger is based on something else, something that's impossible to quantify but easy to describe.

Take my friend Jeannine Trimboli, a personal trainer in New York. Jeannine introduced herself to me on Facebook in March 2010, telling me she was "seeing terrific gains in strength" from Alwyn's program in *NROL for Women*, and "loving" the change in focus. But it wasn't until a year later that she told me what was going on in her life at the time she started lifting heavy. And it was, for lack of a better word, *heavy*.

> Before I read your book, I was a personal trainer who never picked up a weight heavier than 15 pounds. My life at the time was about as low as it could get. I was in the middle of a very messy separation from a very controlling husband, who was fighting me in court. I lost custody of my kids because I was let go from my job. I was alone and scared, a shell of a person.
>
> But something happened as I began lifting heavier weights. I not only got stronger, *I grew a pair of balls*. I fought back. I got custody. I started my own business. I've stopped thinking in terms of what I can or can't do. Now I think about what I *want* to do. And then I do it.
>
> —Jeannine Trimboli, personal trainer, Schenectady, New York

Jeannine is a single mother with four kids. I can say without reservation that she's one of the most sincere individuals I've met in the fitness industry over the past two decades. She wants, more than anything, to help people reach their goals. But first she had to discover a fundamental truth: To help others, she also had to help herself. Pure strength, for her, is empowering. The stronger she got in the gym, the stronger she felt outside of it.

One of the boldest things Jeannine did was post a picture of herself, wearing a bikini at a swimming pool with her kids. Her daughter took the picture when she wasn't looking. The picture showed a strong, athletic physique, with just a hint, if you stared hard enough, of residual mummy tummy. It was about as flat as a human stomach will ever get after giving birth to four children. But it violated an unwritten rule of the fitness industry: You only show skin when you're sure you'll win.

Win what, you ask?

You probably have to spend a lot of time with fitness pros to understand that you're always in competition. With everybody. Whether you want to be or not. Unless you have athletic accomplishments or irrefutable proof of your success with clients, your physique is your business card, your résumé, and your reputation, all rolled into one. (In case you're wondering, I get a pass because of my typing skills.)

The picture brought out the customary trolls, but it sent an even bigger message to women both inside and outside the fitness world: *This is what winning looks like.* It's not just being fit, being healthy, and being strong. It's being comfortable in your own skin. With a big middle finger extended to those with opposing views.

That would be a great place to end the story, except it's not the end.

A year later, while training for her first powerlifting meet, that tiny layer of flesh disappeared. She wasn't trying to get rid of it. It just happened while she focused on something completely different, with higher-intensity workouts and the extra muscle they produced.

Which gives us a convenient opening to talk about the many surprising benefits of training for strength.

MUSCLE DOESN'T WEIGH MORE THAN FAT. BUT IT CAN SURE BEAT THE CRAP OUT OF IT.

When I started writing about fitness, "muscular fitness" and "cardiovascular fitness" were considered two completely separate categories. Separate, and not remotely equal. Cardio fitness, we were told, was the key to health and longevity. You improve cardio fitness by doing endurance exercise, like running, cycling, or rowing. As a bonus, endurance training was also the key to weight loss. The more you do, the thinner you get.

That, as everyone reading this knows, was a powerful incentive for women, then and now. You're bombarded with exhortations to eat less and move more, along with relentless pressure to be thin. And not just thin, but *skinny*. Like a coat hanger, but with straight teeth and blond highlights. Cardio was the only road to that destination.

Lifting? Well, sure, if you want bigger muscles, go ahead and lift. But if you don't also spend hours running or taking aerobics classes, you're SOL, because you've trained your *skeletal* muscles—your arms and shoulders and abs—at the expense of your *cardiac* muscle. Which, we were told, would wither away if it wasn't regularly pumped up with steady-pace endurance exercise. At best you'll leave a well-proportioned corpse, but even that depends on a disciplined, low-fat diet.

And you'll still be dead.

All this seemed so self-evidently obvious that for my first few years in the business, I never heard anyone question it. If you asked which type of exercise burns the most calories, cardio always won. And if you looked around for social proof, again, it was no contest: Runners were sleek and slender. Lifters were thick and lumpy.

Even I believed it, and I had every reason not to. I tried running multiple times (high school, college, late 30s), and with each attempt the same three things happened:

- Saw some improvements
- Stalled out
- Felt worse

Lifting, on the other hand, always made me feel better. The stronger I was, the healthier I felt. And I was, objectively, *healthy*. I stayed lean and felt great without doing any traditional cardio. So while conceding the argument that endurance training does all it's purported to do—burn calories, improve cardiovascular fitness, increase longevity—I always suspected that strength training was undervalued.

And it was. We now know, from a variety of studies, that higher strength is associated with:

- Less body fat
- Less abdominal fat
- Less weight gain over time
- Less risk of diabetes
- Less risk of heart disease
- Less risk of chronic inflammation
- Better outcomes in cancer recovery

Even among teenagers, the strongest girls have less risk of the problems that lead to diabetes and heart disease—high cholesterol, triglycerides, and blood sugar. For older women, strength training preserves the musculoskeletal system—the muscles and bones—that aging whittles away. Put it all together and you get the boss of all benefits:

The strongest women are healthier and live longer, with fewer disabilities.

None of this should be true, based on the conventional understanding of what skeletal muscles are and what they do. They push things. They pull things. They help you pick things up and put them down. They make all human movement possible, and on select individuals they're interesting to look at. But they're basically a lever system, best understood in purely mechanical terms: The biceps pulls on the forearm, which bends the elbow. And that's what little curls are made of.

But if strength training is linked to all the other benefits mentioned, then you have to think there's something else going on. Indeed, there is, and we'll get into that in Chapter 2. First, though, let's define some terms.

WHAT WE MEAN WHEN WE TALK ABOUT STRENGTH

Most of the time, what people call *strength training* doesn't aim to increase strength. The goal is to develop individual muscles, using exercises that allow you to feel those muscles working. So if you do a crunch, you feel a squeeze in your midsection. That squeeze reassures you that you're targeting a problem area. Same with a triceps extension. When you straighten your elbows, you feel a contraction in your triceps, and once again, you think you've done something to improve the appearance of muscles you can see in the mirror, and that others can see when you wear a sleeveless top.

Our approach is different. When Alwyn talks about strength training, he means *training with the goal of getting stronger.* More than that, he means getting stronger by objective standards of strength. There's no objective way to measure your strength on a cable or machine exercise, for example, because there are so many different machines out there. Even the same machine can be calibrated differently in two different gyms.

So when we talk about getting stronger, we look at a handful of basic movement patterns, performed with free weights.

Squat

What it is: For a baby learning to stand upright, the squat is the most natural movement in the world. (It helps not to have bony kneecaps, which typically develop around three years old.) It should be natural for us as well, but becomes less so the older we get and the more time we spend sitting.

Why it matters: Alwyn would never say one exercise is more important than any other. But the squat comes close. Lifting yourself from the bottom position involves all your major lower-body joints and muscles, with active support from your core and torso.

The squat also has the longest paper trail. It's one of three events in the sport of powerlifting, along with the deadlift and bench press, and it's been used for decades in academic research. So while it's hard to link any exercise to direct improvement in any sport, the squat has been correlated with acceleration—takeoff speed—and jumping ability. If all else is equal, the stronger, more explosive athlete should do better in sports like volleyball, softball, basketball, and who knows how many others. Athletes in all sports work to get stronger, and squat strength is almost always one of the ways coaches measure improvements.

The gold-standard measure of strength is the barbell back squat—or, as power-lifters refer to it, the squat. In *NROL for Women*, Alwyn used it in the first workout of the program's first stage. Since then, he's come to see that the barbell squat, with its complex coordination challenges, is a more advanced movement, one that works best when it's preceded by simpler variations like the goblet squat. (I'll get into all this in much more detail in Chapter 13.) You can build meaningful strength in any version, and if this is your first serious training program, you'll amaze yourself when you see what you're capable of lifting.

Deadlift

What it is: You bend forward from the hips and lift a heavy weight off the floor, with most of the force generated by your glutes, your body's biggest and strongest muscles, and your hamstrings. But like the squat, it's really a total-body movement because it starts with the gripping muscles in your hands and forearms and requires strength and stability from almost everything else.

Why it matters: We all have to lift things off the floor. Being able to do it safely will always be useful. But there's more to the deadlift than its practical applications. It has a long and rich history. One of the first recorded feats of strength by a woman was Ivy Russell's 410-pound deadlift in 1930, at a body weight of 134 pounds.

In some ways it's a simpler and better test of strength than the squat. You rarely see anyone in the gym do a competition-depth squat, in which the thighs are slightly below parallel to the floor. More often, lifters shorten their range of motion as they add weight to the bar. But we all have the same idea of what a completed deadlift looks like: You're standing upright, with the weight against your thighs. It's hard to deceive yourself into thinking you lifted something you didn't actually lift.

Pushing Exercises

What they are: You push something away from your body or push your body away from something. We call the latter movement a push-up. The former movement has multiple names, depending on the angle. If you push a weight overhead, we call it a shoulder press. If you're lying on a bench and push a barbell or dumbbells off from your chest, we call it a bench press. If you do that same movement while standing, using a cable machine or elastic band for resistance, we call it a chest press. All these variations use a combination of chest, shoulder, and arm muscles, while the rest of the torso provides stability.

Why they matter: Most of us go into a lifting program with thoughts of how we want specific muscles to look. And as I mentioned at the start of this section, our instinct is to choose exercises that give us immediate feedback, that say, "Yes, those muscles are working."

When you do a push-up, you don't always get that feedback, that sense of specific muscles in action. And that's okay. Muscles are meant to work with each other. Small muscles like the triceps, which straighten your elbow, help the bigger muscles in your chest and shoulders complete the movement. When you add in all the stabilizing muscles that help keep your body straight, it's hard to focus on any one part of the exercise. By the end of the set, if you're working hard, you might be more aware of your breathing than anything else.

It takes some time and effort to figure out if an exercise, or combination of exercises, is doing what you expect. That's why it's so important to focus on strength: As much as you want to trust the process, getting stronger in the major movement patterns is the only way to know for certain that your program is working.

Pulling Exercises

What they are: These are the mirror images of pushing exercises. You pull an object toward your body, as you do in a row or lat pulldown, or pull your body toward an object, as in a chin-up. All of them work the big muscles in your upper and middle back, along with your biceps. Way, way back in our evolutionary history, these were the muscles that allowed our more apelike ancestors to climb trees in search of food or to escape predators.

Why they matter: Everything I said about pushing exercises applies here, as does almost everything I wrote about squats and deadlifts. You may ask what a chin-up has in common with a squat, or a bench press with a deadlift. But in real life, our movements aren't so neatly differentiated.

Imagine, for example, that you're out in public with a toddler. He's normally a happy little guy, but on this day he's a cranky, snot-spewing mess and refuses to get up off the floor of the shopping mall. Somehow you have to lift him from the ground to your shoulder and then carry him, along with a couple of shopping bags and your purse, out to the car.

You may start the process in a full squat (assuming you aren't wearing heels), in order to get enough leverage to lift him from the ground. Raising him to hip level is somewhere between a squat and a deadlift. Hoisting him up and over your shoulder involves the muscles you work in a press, and holding him there is a feat made easier by the muscles trained in chin-ups and rows. The awkwardness of the whole process makes you glad you also did the other exercises in Alwyn's program, including lunges, step-ups, and single-leg movements. And where would you be without all that core-stability training?

Of course it's silly to pretend the goal of a training program is to prepare you for an awkward scenario that humans have been dealing with, in one way or another, as long as humans have existed—lifting, carrying, balancing, moving something from one place to another. The goal of strength training is to look better, move better, and feel better. In the next chapter we'll talk about the muscles that make all that possible and why building them matters.

Why Muscle Matters

When Alwyn and I sat down to talk about *Strong,* my first and biggest question was, what's changed? When you think about training today, how is it different from the way you thought about it in 2006 and 2007, when we wrote *NROL for Women*?

Most of the time, when you ask a trainer that kind of question, you'll get this kind of answer: "I used to think exercise A was the best way to solve problem B, but now we get better results with X, Y, and sometimes Z." Alwyn and I have had lots of conversations over the years about the mechanics of lifting. I always learn something new, and it's always interesting.

This time, though, Alwyn surprised me. "What if we've been wrong about muscle?" he said. Not muscle *training,* but muscle itself. "We've thought about these health benefits as a side effect of training for strength and muscle growth. So you *have* to get stronger, you *have* to get bigger." Otherwise, you don't get anything from the workouts, beyond what you'd get from any type of exercise that burned the same number of calories. "But what if that's completely upside down? What if we looked at muscle as an organ, instead of a lever system? What if strength and muscle growth are side effects of something else?"

Muscle is, in fact, the largest organ system in the human body. For most of us, it accounts for at least 40 percent of our mass. Researchers now think it acts as a "sentinel tissue," predicting the speed and severity of your aging process. Developing the functional ability of your muscles improves your body's defense against the stressors that damage our cells and cause them to age faster than they should.

Another clue that muscle functions as a system: *Just about any method of resistance training will increase muscle strength and size.* This goes against everything Alwyn was taught in graduate school, and everything I learned as a fitness writer. It goes against most of the advice we've received and given. Here's how exercise scientists Stuart Phillips and Richard Winett described the phenomenon in a 2010 review: "Numerous different combinations of resistance, repetitions, and sets produce astonishingly similar, rather than disparate, strength outcomes."

What they all have in common, the authors say, is the degree of effort required to complete a set. It doesn't matter what you lift, or how many times you lift it, as long as you push yourself hard. The harder you work, the more you get out of it. "Resistance simply is a vehicle to produce fatigue," they conclude.

THE FINE PRINT OF MUSCLE TRAINING

Saying muscle is more than a system of levers doesn't mean those levers aren't important. Successful lifters understand the mechanics of lifting, and how to use them to build stronger, higher-quality muscle tissue. I'll start with two interesting data points.

1. **Muscles Start Growing as Soon as You Start Lifting**

   Your strength increases quickly when you begin a new training program. For many years, scientists thought those gains were caused by neural factors—your muscles and nerves learning how to perform new movements—and that actual muscle growth didn't commence for several weeks. We now know that muscle fibers do, in fact, get bigger as you get stronger, no matter if it's your first week of training or your fourth decade. In a study published in the *Journal of Applied Physiology* in 2007, researchers calculated the rate of growth at 0.2 percent per day over the first 20 days of training.

   So while the growth is real, it's minuscule and won't be visually apparent for a long time. (Which explains why it took so long for researchers to detect it.) On the flip side, a novice lifter's first few workouts will create a bit of swelling in and

The Continuum of Effort

Something > Nothing

If there's one thing everyone agrees on, it's that physical activity, in general, is good. Something is always better than nothing, and the biggest benefits are typically seen when a sedentary person gets off her couch and moves. Researchers estimate that regular physical activity, all by itself, increases life expectancy by two to four years. (Women, interestingly, seem to get a greater benefit than men.)

More > Less

You can get additional benefits by doing more, which makes sense. Working out three times a week should be better than once or twice. But each increase in total exercise produces a slightly smaller increase in life-span than the previous increment. So the health benefits of going from two hours of exercise to three hours are more substantial than the additional benefits of going from, say, five hours to six.

Harder > Easier

The maximum boost comes not from doing more work, but by working harder. A review in the *International Journal of Epidemiology* examined three decades' worth of longevity research and concluded that "vigorous exercise and sports" did the most to lower the risk of death from any cause.

Vigorous means you push yourself to at least six times your resting metabolic rate—the amount of energy you expend when you're perfectly still. In exercise science, that state of nonmovement is recorded as 1 metabolic equivalent (MET). Walking around the block is 3 to 4 METs, depending on how fast you go. Running 5 mph (which, for the record, is the best pace I ever managed) is 8 METs. And strength training, according to data compiled in *Medicine & Science in Sports & Exercise*, is 6 METs.

There are two ways to look at that information: You can say, "Running looks better than lifting." If you're talking about total calories burned, you'd be right. Or you could say, "What do they mean by 'strength training'?" Which would be an astute question. There's one way to run—put one foot in front of the other, repeat—and it's relatively straightforward to measure how fast you're going and what happens to your body while you're doing it. But there are many ways to train for strength.

Which is why Alwyn and I wrote this entire book on the subject.

around the muscles, leading some to assume the opposite: *OMG, I'm getting huge!* It's as inspiring for guys as it is terrifying to women. But it means nothing beyond the fact you did something your body wasn't expecting, resulting in mild inflammation.

2.   **The Absolute Amount of Muscle You Can Build Depends on Your Bone Mass**
     The limit for women is 4.2 pounds of muscle tissue per pound of bone. (For men, it's 5 to 1.) You can increase bone thickness by about 1 percent a year through heavy lifting or high-impact competitive sports, which is important but won't substantially increase your upper limit for muscle development. The general size and shape of your frame are set at conception. In other words: *The maximum size of your muscles is determined by your gender and genes.*

This is especially important to remember when the subject of "bulking up" arises. Compared to an average man in the United States, the average woman has about two-thirds as much lean body mass—muscle, bone, and everything else that isn't fat—and two-thirds as much strength. For good measure, she also eats about two-thirds as much food. But the lean mass isn't evenly distributed. Men are typically 40 to 60 percent stronger in the upper body, mostly due to structural issues. My shoulders are naturally wider, support more muscle, and generate more strength and power. (Not that I do anything interesting with it, but that's a different book.) A man's arms carry almost twice as much muscle tissue.

So when we talk about muscle growth, we're talking about a range that starts with what you have now and ends at the limits imposed by the size of your frame. The closer you get to those limits, the harder each incremental improvement will be.

WHAT MAKES MUSCLES GROW

It's actually kind of simple:

1.   Give your muscles a stimulus.
2.   Give your muscles protein.

Your muscles constantly engage in protein turnover, adding new protein to the fibers (synthesis) and shedding the old (breakdown). This occurs every minute of every day, and if you're healthy, should balance itself out in the short term. When you eat a protein-rich meal, there's a brief, transient increase in muscle protein synthesis. And when you lift, synthesis and breakdown both occur at a faster rate; synthesis, in fact, can remain elevated for up to 48 hours. Your goal is to take advantage of this opportunity by giving your muscles plenty of protein, resulting in a net increase.

Protein, which we'll talk about in detail in Chapter 4, is the easy part. For now, let's focus on the stimulus that leads to the desired response: *hypertrophy* (the technical name for muscle growth).

The key to hypertrophy is *mechanical tension*. Challenging your muscles in a workout creates minor disturbances in the structure of their cells. This unleashes a cascade of chemical signals and responses, a process with so many moving parts that even today it isn't fully understood. One of those signals goes to satellite cells. These are stem cells that attach to muscle fibers, giving them more room to add protein.

You can probably think of countless ways to create tension in muscles. Lift something heavy a few times or move something light until your muscles reach a deep state of fatigue or anything in between. Lift a weight as fast as possible or lower it as slowly as you can stand. You can do all this with your own body weight, a barbell, dumbbells, kettlebells, sandbags, bands, or any type of machine. The program can be simple or complicated.

As long as it requires effort, and the effort produces tension, and the tension creates fatigue, and you feed those fatigued muscles, you'll end up with stronger and better-developed muscles, along with a body that's leaner, healthier, and more resistant to stress.

It also goes without saying that your leaner, stronger body will feel better to you and appear more attractive to neutral observers. But it offers one more important benefit, which is the subject of Chapter 3.

3

Why Weight Control (*Not* Weight Loss) Matters

PERHAPS THE GREATEST FRAUD EVER PERPETRATED on American women took root in the early 20th century. It was the idea that no one should gain weight throughout life. Whatever you weighed at age 25 is what you should weigh at 35, 45, 55, and beyond.

To illustrate how insane this is, on the opposite page is an updated version of a chart I put together for *NROL for Life.*

You can see that the average weight of an American woman increased from her 20s to her 30s at every time point in the last half century. Until recently it also increased in the next two decades of life before leveling off among women in their 60s. Weight then declines in the golden years.

If you've reached any of the ages on the right-hand side of the chart, you probably wonder why this is even worth mentioning. *Of course* a woman will gain weight in her 30s. If childbirth doesn't get you, a demanding job will. For many it's a combination of the two. Either way, life in your 30s involves more stress, more responsibility to others, and less time and energy for personal goals like weight management. It takes great effort, great discipline, and/or great genes to weigh the same

AVERAGE WEIGHT FOR ADULT WOMEN IN THE UNITED STATES

Survey Period	Age Range						
	20s	*30s*	*40s*	*50s*	*60–74*	*75+*	
1960–1962	128	139	143	147	147		
1971–1974	134	144	149	148	146		
1976–1980	136	146	149	150	147		
1988–1994	142	154	158	163	154	139	
1999–2002	157	163	168	169	165	147	
					60s	*70s*	*80s*
2003–2006	156	165	171	172	171	156	142
2007–2010	162	169	168	170	171	165	143

Source: National Center for Health Statistics.

at 39 as you did at 25. Hell, *I* packed on some pounds in my late 30s, and all I had to gestate were intestinal flora and perhaps a grudge or two.

Life only gets more demanding in your 40s. And then your reward for meeting all those obligations is menopause.

Human biology is wired to apply the brakes. Without training, we lose about 30 percent of our strength between ages 30 and 60. Lean tissue, including muscle mass, slowly declines and is typically replaced by fat. With less muscle tissue to generate movement, less strength in the muscle we have left, and more fat to carry around, we naturally move less. After all, moving is harder than it used to be.

So when we talk about weight control, it's crucial to frame the conversation in a realistic way. The key points, before we get into the details:

- Almost everyone gains some weight in different stages of life. It's unrealistic to think otherwise.
- If you have a lot of weight you want to lose, for health or aesthetics, you should do exactly that. Nothing in this chapter should be read as an argument in favor of maintaining your current weight if you're not happy with it.
- Weight loss can occur only with a calorie deficit, which you want to create with a combination of diet and exercise. It's like what Alwyn says about progressive-resistance exercise to build strength: It's a law. A written-in-stone law.

But what does that last point even mean? Let's begin there.

ENERGY TO BURN

What we call a "calorie" is actually a *kilocalorie*, which is sometimes abbreviated to *kcal*. One calorie is the energy required to raise 1 gram of water 1 degree Celsius. If that seems bewildering—why are we talking about boiling water?—it's because we don't instinctively think of food as a source of fuel, like gasoline or wood. But that's exactly what it is. When you eat, you fill your body's tank with fuel to keep it running. And it runs all the time, from conception to death. Even when you're asleep your body uses 50 to 75 calories an hour.

At any given moment, you might be in an *energy deficit* (using more calories than you ingest), an *energy surplus* (eating more than you use), or *energy balance* (eating just enough to maintain your current weight).

Where does the energy go when you use it? Into the atmosphere, just like anything else that burns. You can't see it or smell it, but you exhale it all day, every day, in the form of carbon dioxide and water vapor.

The energy comes from a mix of fat (as triglycerides) and carbohydrate (as glucose, aka blood sugar). At rest, a healthy woman burns a little more fat than carbohydrate. During exercise, the ratio reverses, and the harder you work, the more your muscles rely on glucose and the less they rely on fat. But then it shifts again when you stop, and your body burns a higher percentage of fat.

About that fat: We tend to view *dietary fat* and *body fat* as two different things, but it's better to think of them as one thing: a concentrated source of energy, with 9 calories per gram. This is crucial: *Fat is easily and readily used for fuel.* That fuel can come from food or fat cells. Your body doesn't care. It's just fuel.

You probably think of your fat cells as if they're a maximum-security prison. Any fat entering them serves a life sentence with no chance for parole, unless you do something extraordinary, like starve yourself or spend hours a week on a treadmill. Not true. Fat enters and leaves fat cells all the time. The only time you store a significant amount of fat is when you're in a chronic energy surplus. And even then, there's nothing holding the fat in when you shift to an energy deficit. It's an extraordinarily complex chemical process, but so is everything else your body does. The fact that it's complicated doesn't mean your body has a problem with it. It's just one of many metabolic processes your body evolved to do.

Metabolism 101

Technically, *metabolism* means all the chemical processes that occur within and between cells to keep us alive. But when we talk about metabolism, most often we refer to *metabolic rate*, which means the amount of energy our bodies use to perform all the functions of daily life. It has three major components.

THERMIC EFFECT OF FOOD (TEF)

Calories are units of energy, as you know, and through most of human history, it took a lot of energy to procure them—first through hunting, gathering, and scavenging, and eventually through planting, harvesting, and either storing or processing crops. Today, by contrast, it takes a negligible amount of energy to find and prepare food. Even the most elaborate recipe requires less effort to prepare these days than it would've taken centuries ago to turn a bushel of wheat into a loaf of bread or a bucket of milk into a wheel of cheese.

But *digesting* food, no matter how we acquire it, still takes some energy. TEF is usually estimated to be about 10 percent of our daily total. Some foods burn more than others during digestion—protein, the subject of Chapter 4, burns a *lot* more—but no food uses so many calories that it has a negative energy cost. (No, not even celery.)

VOLUNTARY ACTIVITY

Movement you do on purpose, everything from a stroll to the mailbox to a serious workout, will probably make up 20 to 30 percent of your daily calorie burn.

RESTING METABOLIC RATE (RMR)

RMR is your baseline energy expenditure and may account for as much as 70 percent of the total each day. (Your brain alone uses 20 percent of your daily calories.) The rate doesn't shift much from day to day, but over time it can rise and fall, usually because of a change in your lean tissue, which accounts for most of the difference in metabolic rate from one person to the next. Fat, by contrast, uses little energy to sustain itself.

I describe these categories as separate phenomena, but the truth is that they're interrelated. If you eat less, with the goal of losing weight, you burn fewer calories through digestion. You may also move less. Workouts won't be as productive because your body has less energy and may not recover as well from one workout to the next. If you lose lean tissue in the process, your resting metabolism will slow down.

But wait! It gets even worse.

THE SURPRISING CHALLENGES OF WEIGHT LOSS

I keep an email file of all the questions I've answered from readers, going back to 2006. Out of curiosity, I ran a search to see how many contained the phrase *lost weight*. I got more than a hundred matches, which was about 8 percent of the total. A typical question starts like this: "Six months ago, I weighed 200 pounds. Now I weigh 175, and my goal is to get down to 160 by the end of the year." Then the reader describes a grueling workout schedule and disciplined diet plan, and asks what she can add to the workouts or subtract from the diet to attack those final 15 pounds.

My response: Forget about what you haven't lost—for now. Focus instead on the 25 you already dropped. *Make sure those pounds stay lost.* That's every bit as challenging as losing the weight in the first place, and far more important.

Here's why: In weight-loss studies extending a year or more, you often see that participants lose the most weight in the first few months. After the six-month checkpoint, they typically regain a few pounds. There are two mechanisms at work.

Homeostasis

Let's say that in the past year, you ate an average of 1,800 calories a day—typical for an American woman, according to U.S. government data. You didn't eat the exact same amount every day, of course. You had a little less on weekdays, a little more on weekends, and even more on holidays. By the end of the year you probably gained less than a pound. So after eating 657,000 calories spread over 365 days, you may have stored a couple thousand calories altogether. And if you were training throughout the year, some of that stored food is now muscle.

That's how homeostasis works. Your body is extremely good at smoothing out your metabolism to maintain a stable weight. Remember what I mentioned a few paragraphs back: Your RMR doesn't change much from day to day, even though your movement and meals can fluctuate quite a bit. By the end of the year, your body has balanced all those meals and all those workouts to within a few thousand net calories.

It takes something dramatic—like a drop in lean mass—to change your RMR.

Adaptive Thermogenesis

Imagine that you and a friend each weigh 140 pounds. She's been at that weight as long as you've known her. You, on the other hand, recently lost 15 pounds, which was about 10 percent of your original weight. Your new challenge is to maintain your current size. You understand that your leaner, lighter body uses fewer calories per day than it did when you weighed 155 pounds. What you probably haven't considered is that it also uses less energy than your friend's, even though you're equally active and have about the same ratio of fat to muscle.

Studies show that a weight-reduced body has a disproportionately slower resting metabolism. The difference is 136 calories a day in one classic study, a little more in others. A recent study followed a group of men and women for 44 weeks following a brutal crash diet: They ate 500 calories a day for 8 weeks, causing them to shed 10 percent of their weight. By the end of the yearlong experiment, they still showed signs of adaptive thermogenesis, burning 92 fewer calories per day on average.

The exact amount depended on the percentage of weight lost. Those who lost the most, relative to their initial weight, also had the most extreme reaction, while those who regained all their weight by the end of the year returned to their original metabolic rate. The authors of that study, in the bloodless language of research, say the reduction "may predispose to weight regain." To which you might respond, "Ya *think*?"

Once again, there's a diabolical efficiency at work. Even if you don't like what it does, you have to at least appreciate the complexity of it. Once you do that, you might ask a more difficult question: If *you* want to lose weight, why does your body resist? Who's in charge here?

WHY "NORMAL WEIGHT" IS NEITHER NORMAL NOR IDEAL

The abundance of food we enjoy today is almost unprecedented in our history. Even in the recent past, if someone lost weight it was probably unintentional, the result of disease, natural calamity, or a run of extremely bad luck. To put that in contemporary language: "I need to lose some of this flesh so I can fit into my skinny furs," said no Paleolithic woman ever.

But that was then. Today, a typical article about weight loss will begin with a sentence like this: "Almost 70 percent of American adults are overweight or obese."

The category of "overweight" refers to anyone with a body mass index (BMI) of 25 or more. That includes me. I'm 5 foot 10, and when I weigh myself in the morning, I'm usually between 176 and 178 pounds. That puts my BMI just over 25. A woman who's 5 foot 4 and 147 pounds is right there with me—slightly overweight, according to BMI. (To check your own, just type "BMI calculator" into a search engine, and you'll have plenty to choose from.) At 180 pounds, she'd be "obese," with a BMI just over 30.

BMI is an extremely crude measure of health because it doesn't account for how your body looks or what it can do. It's useful for population studies, but not for individuals like you or me. What you may not know is that BMI wasn't used to determine who was or wasn't overweight until the early 1980s. Before that, we used words like "ideal," "desirable," "acceptable," or "suggested" to describe the weight that, according to the actuarial tables of life-insurance companies, was associated with the lowest risk of death from any cause.

By today's standards, the tables were comically random. People applying for life insurance were often allowed to report their own height and weight. Men, being men, would exaggerate their height, and women, being women, would underreport their weight. The current cutoff points—a BMI over 25 is "overweight," and anything over 30 is "obese"—date all the way back to 2000. More important, while some earlier standards acknowledged that adults over 35 tend to be heavier than younger ones, the new cutoff points apply to *everybody*. We're back to the crazy idea that no one should ever gain weight.

I can't tell you what the practical result of all this is. Do doctors advise their patients to lose weight, based on BMI? A doctor once told me I need to, but at the time I actually agreed with him. (I eventually took off about 10 pounds.) Most Americans, when asked, will tell researchers and pollsters that they'd like to lose weight, which suggests that most Americans understand they're heavier than they should be, according to other Americans.

And yet it's impossible to say what the ideal weight is for any of us. To repeat: *No one knows the healthiest weight for you at any point in your life.*

Katherine Flegal understands this as well as anyone. As an epidemiologist for the Centers for Disease Control and Prevention, she more or less discovered the obesity epidemic in the early 1990s and has done much of the data crunching since then. Flegal created a stir in 2013 when she ran the numbers on body weight and mortality and found, to the surprise of many, that people who're technically overweight live longer than those in the "normal weight" category.

Their extra body mass, it seems, is protective, particularly against the ravages of age and wasting diseases. Heavier people fare better in car accidents, surgery, and cancer treatment. And they're less likely to get lung cancer or to fall and break a hip.

The difference isn't huge, and it certainly doesn't mean we should start advising people to *gain* weight. But it's real. It's been found in too much credible research across too many medical disciplines to be a fluke.

So what does it mean?

Fat mass, aesthetics aside, may offer a few basic advantages—a cushion in high-speed accidents, some margin of error against horrible diseases—but comes with a long list of disadvantages. The heavier you are, the more risk there is of cardiovascular and musculoskeletal problems, and all the other things the Internet will gladly warn you about.

But lean mass, the kind you build in the weight room and use in any type of physical activity, offers nothing but advantages.

THE HAMMER OF THE GODDESSES

One of my favorite articles for *Men's Health* had nothing specifically to do with men. It started with an editorial published in an obscure exercise science journal that asked an intriguing question: What if the entire basis of weight-loss research is wrong? It arose when the author Bernard Gutin began a long-term study of several hundred teenagers in 2000. The goal was to see how exercise and diet influenced risk factors for cardiovascular disease. Gutin and his colleagues went into the project with the simple, uncontroversial idea that the kids who ate the most would be the fattest and at greatest risk for health problems down the road.

But that's not what they found. Instead, the kids who ate the most were the leanest. They weren't the *lightest*, but they had the lowest body-fat percentages in the study. Even more interesting: They weren't necessarily exercising more than the less-lean kids. What separated the leanest was *vigorous* exercise. They did more running, jumping, and lifting. They played more sports. As a result, they had more lean tissue and less fat, despite eating more than the fattest kids in the study.

That seemed impossible to Gutin, who's been around so long he's an emeritus professor at two different universities. It was enough to make him rethink the most basic premise of weight-loss advice: If you're fat, it's because you ate too much. What if the problem isn't overeating, he asked, but undertraining?

Now, we're all adults in this room, and as adults we can admit that weight control is too complex for an either-or question. For a physique that's better than the one you have now, you need some combination of diet and training. The only question up for debate is whether you've focused too much on the calories you consume and not enough on the calories you burn and how you burn them. Your answer to that question will be different from mine or anyone else's. A few things you should know:

People Who Train More Also Eat More

Weight-loss advice inevitably exhorts you to "eat less and move more," which Alwyn describes as "one of the most absurd statements in history." How can you demand more of a body when you're giving it less to work with? You may think there's good research behind this idea, but there's not. In the long-running Women's Health Study, for example, the middle-aged women who did the most exercise also ate the most and were least likely to gain weight during a 12-year period.

Lean Mass Increases Your Metabolism, and a Faster Metabolism Increases Your Appetite

Compare the RMR of any two people (you and me, you and your mom, your mom and me . . .) and lean mass will explain about 50 to 60 percent of the difference. Fat tissue will account for 5 to 6 percent. Age and gender have at most a minor effect. My bones, muscles, and organs are probably bigger than yours, which makes my metabolism faster. If your bones, muscles, and organs are bigger than your mom's, your metabolism will be faster.

Research at the University of Leeds in England shows that RMR drives appetite, including the total amount of food you eat in a day and the size of individual meals. The higher your metabolic rate, the hungrier you'll be. So adding a few pounds of muscle will indeed make you at least a bit hungrier from meal to meal and day to day.

Luckily, there's a simple way to manage that hunger and make it work for you, rather than thwart your goals: eat more protein and less of everything else.

Why Protein Is the Key to a Successful Diet

THE WORD *PROTEIN* COMES FROM THE Greek *proteios*, meaning "first rank" or "most important." Dutch biochemist Gerhard Mulder was the first to use it in a scientific context. I won't try to describe what he *thought* he'd discovered when he gave it that awesome name back in 1838, mostly because I don't understand it. All I can say for certain is that the name stuck while the definition changed. What we now call protein is one of the three macronutrients, along with fat and carbohydrate. We know it helps with weight control in three hugely important ways:

- It helps us build and maintain lean tissue. Muscle, once you drain the water, is almost entirely made of protein.
- It has a higher thermic effect than carbs or fat. About 25 percent of protein calories are used during digestion, compared to 6 to 8 percent for carbs and 2 to 3 percent for fat.
- It helps you feel full faster during a meal, and helps you go longer between meals before you feel hungry again.

Add those three features up, and you get a result that's been shown over and over in weight-loss research: People who are assigned to eat more protein lose more fat, retain more muscle, have less hunger, and eat less total food. In animal studies, lower protein typically leads to overeating, fat gain, and muscle loss. This has led some scientists to suggest that all animals, including humans, "leverage" protein. That is, through unknown mechanisms, we keep track of how much protein we've eaten, and this tracking system helps regulates our appetite. We eat more food when we have less protein in our meals, and less when we have more. In other words, hunger is really a quest for protein.

The protein-leverage hypothesis made intuitive sense to me. One of the great paradoxes of our affluent culture is that the wealthiest people are the leanest, and the poorest are the fattest. Because protein tends to be expensive, the cheapest food has the least protein, and the protein it has tends to be of the lowest quality. (One study found that fast-food hamburgers are only about 12 percent meat; the rest is mostly water, with bits and pieces of cartilage and bone ground into the mix.) You can see the problem: If all you eat is low-quality, mass-produced food, you'll probably need a lot more of it to reach your body's internal protein target. A diet of cheap, crappy food will make you bigger and fatter. The bigger you are, the more there is to feed, which means you'll need even more protein and eat even more cheap, crappy food to attain it.

In a terrific book called *The Nature of Nutrition: A Unifying Framework from Animal Adaptation to Human Obesity*, authors Stephen Simpson and David Raubenheimer show that, for most species, the leverage effect kicks in when 15 percent of the calories in the diet come from protein.

But so far, it doesn't seem to work that way in humans. For starters, the average American gets about 15 percent of her calories from protein already. Another complication: There are 20 amino acids, the building blocks of protein, and there are countless ways to combine and configure them. Does your body treat all those combinations the same or does it have a unique reaction to each? Then you have myriad combinations of fat, carbohydrate, fiber, vitamins, and minerals in protein-rich foods. Does your body react the same way to the protein in a fatty T-bone steak as it does to a lean chicken breast? What about the protein in beans, milk, soy, eggs, nuts, or seafood?

When researchers have tried to detect protein leverage in clinical experiments, they find it seems to occur only when protein makes up 30 percent of total calories. That's when the men and women in the studies ate less and experienced less overall hunger. No surprise there; lots of studies have shown similar results.

In one meta-analysis—a compilation of the results of multiple studies into one pool of data—researchers examined 24 weight-loss studies that compared higher-protein diets (25 to 35 percent of total calories) with standard-protein diets (12 to 18 percent); study participants ate the same amount of fat and total calories. Individuals who ate more protein lost 1 pound more, on average, over a variety of durations, from a month to a year.

One pound doesn't sound like much, until you consider that the subjects ate the same amount of food. Those eating more protein not only lost slightly more weight but also improved their body composition by gaining a small amount of muscle (even without an exercise program) and losing more fat than those eating less protein.

You can guess why more protein worked better:

- More muscle means a higher resting metabolic rate (an average of 142 calories a day in the studies that measured it).
- More protein means more calories burned during digestion.
- More protein means greater satiation from a meal (that is, you feel full faster) and a longer gap before feeling hungry again.

And there's one way to get even more out of a higher-protein diet.

PROTEIN + STRENGTH TRAINING = MUSCLE

No one can tell you the perfect amount of protein to eat for your goals. I'm biased toward higher amounts because (1) we know they help you build and retain more muscle, and (2) the more you eat, the lower your appetite for everything else. So, with that in mind, let's run through a few basic recommendations.

How Much?

Suppose you're a typical lifter who trains relatively hard four hours a week: three hours in the gym and another hour of cardio. You weigh 130 pounds. Your goals are to get stronger and improve your body composition—the ratio of fat to lean tissue—without gaining or losing weight. You won't *complain* if you lose a couple of pounds, but it's not your focus right now.

First let's get a simple and unscientific approximation of your daily energy needs.

We'll take your current weight and multiply it by 10. That gives us 1,300 calories a day, a very crude approximation of your resting metabolism. Then we'll add your weight multiplied by 4, to represent four weekly hours of training. If you were writing it as an equation, it would look like this:

$$130 \times (10 + 4) = 1{,}820 \text{ calories}$$

That, in theory, represents the energy you'd need each day to maintain your current weight with your current workout schedule. Your actual needs could be higher or lower, and if your goal was to lose weight, you'd probably want to start with your *target weight*, rather than your current size. But let's go with your present weight for now.

A standard recommendation is to eat 2 grams of protein per kilogram of body weight. To get your weight in kilograms, we do this: 130 lb ÷ 2.2 = 59 kg. So

$$2 \times 59 = 118 \text{ grams of protein per day}$$

Protein has 4 calories per gram; 118 grams is 472 calories from protein per day, which is 26 percent of your daily calories. As I said, there's no precise formula to predict the perfect amount for you. And in truth, there's probably no such thing as "perfect." Your body can thrive with lots of different combinations of macronutrients. Our best guess is that 25 to 35 percent of your daily calories will probably give you all the benefits you can get from protein, while leaving plenty of room for everything else; between two-thirds and three-quarters of your daily calories will be fat and carbs.

How you allocate those calories is entirely a matter of personal preference. In weight-loss studies, lower-carb diets tend to get better results in the first few months. But once you go 12 months or longer, the percentage of carbs and fat doesn't matter nearly as much as individual adherence—how closely you follow the plan. And what makes you stick with a diet? Personal preference, right? You have to like the food.

When?

Let's start with a visualization: To get 118 grams of protein in one meal, you could eat

- 20 eggs
- 4.2 cups of cottage cheese
- 4 cups of soybeans
- 14 ounces of chicken (2 large breasts)
- 1.3 pounds of salmon

- 22 ounces of bacon
- 8 cups of black beans

These examples are absurd, which is the point. The best way to eat a lot of protein in a day is to spread it out across multiple meals. Researchers at Skidmore College have published several studies on the benefits of timed protein intake. In one, they had volunteers eat six meals a day, each with about 20 grams of protein. The meals were evenly spaced, so the participants had the first one as soon as they woke up, the last one shortly before bedtime, and the others at three-hour intervals. They concluded that you do get a benefit from eating six meals a day, compared to three, and from eating protein at three-hour intervals.

It makes sense to me, but that's in part because I'm a lifelong breakfast eater who does better with four or five smaller meals than with two or three bigger ones. But is it the best way for *you* to eat? A few years ago I would've said yes, because breakfast is the most important meal of the day, blah blah blah. Now we know that different people thrive with different meal patterns and eating styles.

But there is one *crucial* timing question.

POST-WORKOUT?

In previous books, including *NROL for Women*, my coauthors and I emphasized the importance of the post-workout "window of opportunity." We know our muscles break down and synthesize protein at a faster rate after training. A post-workout dose takes advantage of that phenomenon to build muscle while minimizing breakdown. The maximum effective dose is said to be 20 grams (which is why the aforementioned research team used that amount in their studies), which is a single scoop of a typical protein supplement. Older lifters probably need more; one study of older men showed that it took 40 grams to max out protein synthesis. Since the men were in their 70s, it's impossible to know how this applies to a 50-year-old woman, or anyone in between.

But here's an important question: If your body is almost always in the process of recovering from your most recent workout, and you habitually eat several protein-rich meals a day, how important is that post-workout protein infusion? Some researchers say it still matters, while others say it doesn't if you eat within a couple hours before and after your workouts.

For Alwyn, there's no question: He's 100 percent in favor of post-workout protein. "I think it falls into the 'might help, *definitely* won't hurt' category," he told me.

"As a trainer, I can't make sure a client eats a perfect breakfast or lunch. *Maybe* she'll leave the gym, go home, and have grilled chicken, rice, and vegetables. If she does, *maybe* she'll get the same benefits.

"Unfortunately, there's just as good a chance that life will get in the way, and she'll miss her next meal. There's a chance she'll get home and find nothing in the fridge. There's also a chance she missed the previous meal, too.

"But I can hand her a shake with 20 grams of whey protein and fruit. And now we're both sure.

"I can't think of a single reason why my client's results would improve if she skipped that post-workout shake in favor of something she may or may not eat later."

Alwyn makes one final point: "After one of these workouts, I can assure you that a plate of salmon and asparagus is *not* an exciting prospect."

Why not? Several classic studies have shown something Alwyn knows from many years of experience: Intense exercise temporarily lowers appetite. There doesn't seem to be any long-term effect, which makes sense, based on what we covered in Chapter 3. If you're training hard enough to build muscle and raise your resting metabolic rate, of course you're going to eat a little more. But immediately after one of his workouts? An ice-cold protein shake, sweetened with some fruit, should hit the spot.

What?

I mentioned that there are 20 amino acids. Of those, leucine is by far the most important for building muscle. Maximum protein synthesis is thought to occur with 1.5 grams of leucine. The chart opposite (a self-share from *Supercharged*) shows how different foods have widely different leucine concentrations.

As you can see, there are lots of ways to get 20 grams of protein and 1.5 grams of leucine in a single serving of a single food. (The ones in bold have the highest leucine concentration.) Just about any normal serving of meat or fish will do the trick. According to the Internet, 3 ounces is about the size and thickness of a deck of cards, a bar of soap, or the palm of your hand; most of the portions shown in the chart are just a little bigger than that.

Personally, I like the convenience of supplements, and after decades of use in research, it's clear they do the one thing we want them to do: get protein to the muscles as quickly as possible. Most supplements used in studies are made from milk proteins. Milk is 80 percent casein and 20 percent whey, but supplements are typically made from whey isolate. Some recent research shows that whey supple-

Food Source	Serving Size	Protein, grams	Leucine, grams
Almonds	¼ cup	6.6	0.5
Beef (sirloin)	4 ounces	21	1.6
Black beans	1 cup	15	1.2
Chicken	**½ breast**	**30**	**2.2**
Corn	1 cup	5	0.5
Cottage cheese	**1 cup**	**28**	**2.9**
Eggs	3 whole	18	1.6
Greek yogurt	1 cup	20	1.6
Lentils	1 cup	16	1.3
Milk, 2 percent	2 cups	16	1.6
Mozzarella cheese	3 ounces	16	1.6
Oats	½ cup	13	1
Peanut butter	2 tablespoons	8	0.7
Pork loin	5 ounces	20	1.6
Salmon	4 ounces	23	1.8
Soybeans	**1 cup**	**29**	**2.3**
Whey-protein supplement*	**1 scoop**	**20**	**2**
Whole-wheat bread	2 slices	5	0.4
Wild rice	½ cup	11	0.8

Source: *Nutrition Almanac*, 6th ed.

* I used Biotest Low-Carb Metabolic Drive, which I had on hand.

ments are useful in treating symptoms of type 2 diabetes, although it's not clear if those benefits derive from protein in general or one specific type.

I know supplements aren't for everybody, for various reasons. Cost, obviously, comes into play. Some people don't like using supplements on principle, often because they don't trust the industry to provide safe and effective products. I don't share that distrust, but I understand it.

For vegans, soy isolates appear to be a good choice, and as of this writing, soy is the only type that's been compared directly to whey in strength-training research. Those studies show no difference in muscle hypertrophy over 6 to 12 weeks. I don't know of any exercise research that looks at other vegetarian proteins, like hemp.

Before we move on to the training program, there's one more topic I want to tackle.

Why All This Still Seems So Confusing

For most of human civilization, people who feel called to provide authoritative information—teachers, writers, doctors—have been frustrated by the public's stubborn refusal to pay attention. In head-to-head competition, rigorous scholarship loses almost every round to superstition and rumor. You can guess why: Gossip and folk wisdom are based on what we suspect or want to believe is true. It's correct just often enough to support our faith in our own common sense and intuition.

Take the story of my friend Brynda Ivan. In November 1997, she was 30 years old and 50 pounds overweight. She'd tried lots of interventions, but none had clicked. Then she went to her first Weight Watchers meeting, and for reasons she can't explain, she decided to follow through. She lost 50 pounds in a year and managed to establish a regular exercise routine—first walking, then running. "But I still had no clue how to exercise effectively or maintain lean mass," she told me.

She joined a fitness center near her home, where a trainer showed her how to use the machines and told her to do 10 reps on each one. It didn't take long to realize the limitations of that program. "I started reading magazines and books about exercise," she said. "I took kickboxing classes and step aerobics classes. I spent hours on the StairMaster and elliptical machines. Every magazine and book told me something different, and I jumped from one thing to the next. One magazine told me to do cardio for 'toning.' The next magazine told me to lift, but be sure to keep the weights light or risk getting bulky. The next told me to stick to machines or risk serious injury. Eventually I found some bodybuilding-style workouts in a magazine. Isolate each muscle, work it in a fixed plane."

She still cringes at the memories.

I know Brynda because she eventually discovered *NROL for Women*, developed a passion for squats and deadlifts, and found an online community of fellow enthusiasts. Now she's a regular at the annual Fitness Summit in Kansas City, where I act as emcee, and we keep in touch year-round.

Brynda is probably a lot like you: smart, competent, well-educated, and well-informed. But because she lacked a background in exercise science, every source of information appeared just as credible to her as any other.

Start with the most traditional way to communicate knowledge: from master to apprentice, and from apprentice to novice. That was especially true within gym culture, where it was assumed that a person who's extremely strong and/or muscular must know what he's talking about. It's still the best way to learn the fundamentals; just about every great lifter or coach I've met has a story about an influential mentor. But it's also a great way to perpetuate misinformation, including what we now call "broscience." A few representative nuggets:

- Muscle that's left untrained will turn to fat.
- Fat can be turned into muscle.
- Muscle soreness means you had a good workout.

Maybe you already know that muscle can't become fat and that no alchemy can turn fat to muscle. And maybe you know muscle soreness is a sign you did something *different* in your workout, but not necessarily better or worse—it all depends on the context.

Or maybe you didn't know, but wonder why it matters. If you train hard to reach your goals, who cares if you misunderstand the process?

It matters because of a closely related type of advice: guru science. It's guided by a logic that goes something like this: "Expert A trains Celebrity B. Celebrity B looks awesome. Therefore, Expert A must know what he's talking about." Expert A then morphs into a guru by offering extremely specific advice to his celebrity clients, and sharing bits and pieces of it with the public:

- Eating *this* food at *this* time will make you fat (bonus points for naming the hormones responsible for this calamity).
- Doing an exercise in *this* way (instead of *that* way) will produce *this* change in the shape of the targeted muscle.
- Ingesting *these* supplements at the beginning/middle/end of your workout will give you a benefit you can't get by doing the same things in any other sequence.

Exercise and nutrition scientists know it's highly unlikely that any of these details matter as much as the guru implies. Your body is too complex for that. If you're new to strength training, your muscles will be breaking down and synthesizing protein at a faster than normal rate for 24 to 48 hours after a workout. (It's more like 16 hours for an experienced lifter.) *All* the food you eat matters, not just what you take in at designated moments. That said, it's possible, and perhaps even likely, that specific rules and rituals help the guru's clients bring order to otherwise chaotic lives. But for most of us, they make exercise and nutrition more complicated than they need to be.

Somewhere in between broscience and guru science is femscience. My coauthors and I did our best to debunk two of the prime examples in *NROL for Women*:

- Lifting heavy weights will give you thick, bulky muscles.
- Using light weights for high reps will give you long, lean, toned muscles.

As we argued, very few women have the genetic potential to put on a lot of muscle. Even for guys, it's much harder than any of us expect when we start out. I'm happy to say we've made some inroads on the bulking vs. toning front. But it wasn't science that won the argument. It was experience. Women who tried heavy lifting loved the results. Not all, certainly, but enough to make a difference.

Alas, coaches like Alwyn and writers like me are powerless against the two founding principles of femscience:

- To lose fat, you must emphasize cardio over strength training.
- To lose fat in "problem areas," you must do specialized exercises for those areas.

The "every woman needs to do aerobic exercise" tenet remains because almost every woman has been convinced she needs to lose weight. That's a societal phenomenon, with persistence beyond the power of reason or argument.

The idea of spot reducing, on the other hand, should be banished by now. We have plenty of research showing that no exercise can selectively target isolated pockets of fat. But no matter how hard the fitness industry pushes back, it's subtly reinforced in articles, books, and training programs that promise to "sculpt a sexy" this or a "toned" that. They won't come right out and say "this exercise burns fat from that place where you don't want it," but they certainly imply it.

There's one more belief that links femscience, broscience, and guru science with popular culture: "If I do the workout of Celebrity X, I can get arms/legs/earlobes like Celebrity X." You've seen this myth promoted over and over, especially on the covers of checkout-line magazines.

The truth, of course, is that you can't change the shape of your muscles. You can only make them bigger or allow them to atrophy. With a solid training program, like Alwyn's, you can also reduce fat systemically. But you have no control over what your individual parts look like when you're in top shape. All you know is that you'll almost certainly look and feel better than you did before.

Finally, there's a type of information that isn't based on fiction or wishful thinking. Sometimes it begins as real science. But that doesn't mean it's accurate.

OLD SCIENCE

My friends with advanced degrees like to say that science has no expiration date. And of course that's true, in the sense that research published in respected journals, and not subsequently retracted, provides timeless information. It tells us what scientists thought was worth investigating at that time, how they approached the problem, and what they found.

Scientific knowledge, however, is like the universe itself: always in motion and constantly expanding. Important questions are never settled with a single experiment. That's why most of the research I cite in the notes was published within two or three years of the period when Alwyn and I wrote *Strong*. Where I used older studies, I was confident the results hadn't been contradicted by more recent findings. (In some cases I know or have at least corresponded with the studies' authors.)

I also, when appropriate, try to use review studies, especially meta-analyses, which combine the results of multiple experiments to create a larger pool of data.

My final safeguard is my own judgment. Some research groups have longer and more substantial track records, and from following their work over the years, I'm confident they ask the right questions and seek answers with appropriate rigor.

Still, it's impossible to be 100 percent evidence based, 100 percent of the time. We often default to conventional wisdom, even if we don't know where it originated. A few examples:

- Breakfast is the most important meal of the day.
- It's better to eat four to six small meals a day instead of two or three big ones.
- A pound of muscle burns an extra 50 calories a day.
- We need eight glasses of water a day to avoid dehydration.

Some are based on correlations—people who do something (like eat small meals, including a daily breakfast) are lighter and/or leaner than people who don't. The wildly optimistic estimate of muscle's effect on your metabolism was probably a misinterpretation of older research. And I'm not sure if anyone knows how we arrived at eight glasses of water as some kind of magic number. (It may come from a 1945 U.S. government publication, leaving off the part that said most of your daily water will come from food.)

Sometimes even when science is correct, it's more nuanced than we've been told. Here's an example:

In just about any weight-loss article or fitness book, including my own, the author will mention that a pound of fat contains 3,500 calories of energy. That much is true. But it's usually followed by something like this: "If you cut 500 calories a day from your diet, you'll lose a pound of fat every week." It doesn't work like that in real life.

A 2013 study in the *International Journal of Obesity* looked at actual vs. predicted weight loss in studies in which every aspect of the subjects' lives was controlled and every calorie of food was accounted for. Using the 3,500-calories-per-pound rule, they should've lost 27 percent more weight than they actually did.

Kevin Hall, an obesity and metabolism researcher at the National Institutes of Health, calculates that it really takes a deficit of 4,300 calories to lose a pound of fat. But even that is inconsistent. Leaner people lose weight faster than those with a higher body fat percentage, and men lose faster than women. That's with the exact same reduction in calories.

Another complication: All weight loss includes a combination of fat and lean tissue. But it takes a deficit of only 828 calories to lose a pound of muscle. Since lean tissue drives your metabolism, any change in one will also change the other. That's in addition to the fact that you'll burn fewer calories during digestion when you eat less food.

So where does this leave us? If broscience, femscience, and guru science are so often wrong, and the conventional wisdom is so often outdated, and even scientists who specialize in weight loss may not fully appreciate how complex it is, what's a normal woman with a busy life to do? Whom can you rely on?

THE HIERARCHY OF EXPERTISE

Sorting through conflicting claims by genuine experts is a tough challenge for non-experts. It's made even tougher by the fact that anyone can look like an expert. All it takes is a few big words and some footnotes. So what's a busy person to do?

1. **If It's Life and Death, Trust the Experts**

    Don't try to second-guess the paramedic when you're bleeding out. And when the doctor is putting your fractured arm back together, that's not really the time to ask if the bandage was made from genetically modified cotton.

2. **For Basic Health and Longevity, the Conventional Wisdom Is Probably Good Enough**

    You don't have to become an expert on every topic related to health, fitness, or nutrition. The best insurance we have against premature disability or death is to stay active and practice moderation in all things. Work hard, but not too hard. Get sleep, but not too much. Exercise, but not to extremes. Enjoy the good things in life, but not too many of them at the same time. The specifics—what type of work you do, how you exercise, what you eat—aren't all that important.

3. **For Advanced Results, You Need Someone with Specialized Knowledge**

    If you walked into a fitness conference and saw all the speakers lined up, it's unlikely you'd be able to figure out who specializes in what. You certainly wouldn't look at Alwyn and assume he's an expert in fat loss. When I first met him in the late 1990s, I thought of him as a generalist, same as most of the trainers I knew back then. His reputation grew out of that general practice, when the methods he used to help clients get bigger and stronger also helped them get leaner. It's an important insight he might not have gained had he set out to specialize in fat loss, especially at a time when that meant focusing on cardio and a low-fat, low-calorie diet.

That's the interesting thing about genuine expertise: It often emerges from unique circumstances in which the expert found himself or herself in the right place at the right time with the right knowledge, skills, and ambition to take advantage of the opportunity. The individual may be a highly educated professional, a high school dropout, or anything in between, and the specialization may or may not be what he or she set out to do. What matters is the evidence, the success of the expert's athletes or students or clients. This is especially important to remember at a time when anybody with a URL can claim to be a "world-renowned" specialist in one thing or another. A genuine expert can back it up.

BEWARE THE RABBIT HOLES OF THE INTERNET

But what if you're not satisfied with these choices and decide to develop your own expertise? I know exactly how you feel. I spent my first few years as a fitness journalist doing what I'd been trained to do—interviewing experts and acting as a conduit from them to our readers. It didn't take me long to figure out the limits of that approach: Unless I became an expert myself, I couldn't tell the difference between good advice and guru-science bullshit. So I took classes, studied textbooks, earned personal-trainer certifications, and did what I could to learn what experts knew, and by extension to think the way they did about their areas of expertise. I'm still a journalist, but I'm also a fitness professional with more than two decades' worth of experience.

In the process, I found that the more I learned, the more I wanted to learn. Which is great, except for the times when each Internet search took me further down the same path. For me, it's merely a waste of energy. But for someone who may be exploring a subject for the first time, what at first seems like a rabbit hole can become a giant vacuum that sucks you in and never lets you out.

It starts innocently enough: You come across an idea that makes sense. It tells you something you want to believe. Maybe it's presented as information that's been denied to you by a rigidly conformist establishment. Soon you're reading only the work of people with a single point of view. The further you go, the more that point of view shifts from advocacy of one thing to opposition to everything else. What started as a community morphs into a cult, with its own code words and group identity. Those with the most passion and time on their hands create an inner circle of true believers, who take it upon themselves to codify and then enforce their belief system. Winning arguments becomes more important than finding new ways to solve the problems that brought the group together in the first place. Doubters become dissenters. Dissenters become apostates. Splinter groups form. Friendships shatter. Wars are declared, and it's only a matter of time before Oceania invades Eastasia.

I'm just kidding about the invasion. But the rest has happened over and over. Diets, exercise systems, and health interests eventually bring out the worst, most tribal instincts in our fellow humans. Even the people who pride themselves on being dispassionate and evidence oriented can sometimes become *militantly* dispassionate and evidence oriented, sneering with moral superiority and hurling their peer-reviewed citations like acid into the eyes of the less informed.

And that, to the consternation of our editors, is my segue to the heart and soul of *Strong*: Alwyn's training programs. Alwyn, as I noted, started as a generalist. He tests new tools and techniques when they come along, and integrates the ones that work into his programs. But he never goes all-in on the fad of the moment. Nor does he forget that what worked before the latest thing came along still works.

So. Are you ready to do this thing?

PART 2

The Training Program

6

How the System Works

ALWYN'S SYSTEM HAS NINE STAGES, EACH of which is a distinct workout program that builds on the strength and skill you attain in the previous stage. We group these programs into three phases:

Phase One: Develop (Chapter 7)

The three programs in Phase One, Stages 1 to 3, are a fresh start for everyone. For a beginner, of course, anything is a fresh start. But all of us can benefit from a return to basic exercises and methods. If you've been lifting for years, you may have lost some of the qualities you initially developed. For example, if you never do high-rep sets, you can lose muscular endurance. Same with basic core stability, if you've stopped doing exercises like planks and side planks. If you've emphasized your strengths in the weight room while ignoring the things you don't love as much—and who doesn't want to focus on what they like and do well?—there's a good chance you've trained your way into imbalances, with disproportionate strength in one movement pattern or set of muscles. Phase One helps you restore what was lost or was perhaps never developed to begin with.

After you complete all the workouts in Stage 1, you'll do the Special Workout, which calls for a single all-out set of seven key strength exercises, using the same weights (or variations, in the case of the body-weight exercises) you used in the second workout of Stage 1. The obvious purpose is to demonstrate how much stronger you are just two to three weeks later. But the covert goal is to show you how much you held back with the weights you selected in your early workouts. That should give you the confidence to be more aggressive in the next part of the program.

Phase Two: Demand (Chapter 8)

You'll be glad you went back to basics, because in Phase Two you'll build on everything you developed or restored in Phase One. The exercises are more advanced, and the system—which includes a higher-intensity technique that will be new to most readers—is more complex.

Phase Three: Display (Chapter 9)

Now we get to the part that some of you will be tempted to start with—which, of course, we discourage. The workouts in Phase Three push you to your limits, with the goal of setting performance standards that you may never exceed. The more preparation you have, the better those all-time-best numbers will be.

PROGRAM BASICS

In most stages, you'll have two total-body workouts—Workout A and Workout B— which you'll alternate until you've done each of them four to six times. Because these are complete workouts, you'll never do A and B on the same day. Nor should you do them on consecutive days.

You'll have the most success if you lift three times a week, with at least one day off in between workouts. Two strength workouts a week can also work, especially if you're playing a sport or training for another fitness goal. (We'll give you specific tips in Chapter 15.) Opposite is how a month of workouts might look if you train three times a week, using a standard Monday-Wednesday-Friday schedule.

As you can see, if you do each workout six times—12 total workouts—it'll take you four weeks to complete a stage. In Phase One, the more advanced or impatient lifters can move on after doing each workout four times. Everyone will do each of the Phase Two workouts six times, and in Phase Three you'll do each one four times.

	Monday	Tuesday	Wednesday	Thursday	Friday	Saturday	Sunday
Week 1	Workout A	off	Workout B	off	Workout A	off	off
Week 2	Workout B	off	Workout A	off	Workout B	off	off
Week 3	Workout A	off	Workout B	off	Workout A	off	off
Week 4	Workout B	off	Workout A	off	Workout B	off	off

WHAT YOU DO

Each workout has the following elements:

RAMP (Chapter 11)

Put most simply, RAMP is a warm-up. That is, it gets your body warm and ready to lift heavy things. It's also a sophisticated way to, as the acronym says, increase your range of motion, activate muscles, and employ movement preparation. If you've read *Abs*, *Life*, and/or *Supercharged*, you're familiar with the principles. The exercises change as Alwyn tweaks his protocols, but the goal of developing and then maintaining optimal mobility remains constant.

Core Training (Chapter 12)

Core training includes one, two, or sometimes three exercises designed to target the muscles that support the lower back and pelvis. The combination of RAMP and core training usually takes me 15 minutes, but if all the exercises are new to you, it'll take a little longer.

Strength Training (Chapters 13 and 14)

Each workout in Phase One and Phase Two has four strength exercises. (The Phase Three workouts are structured differently, as you'll see in Chapter 9.) A typical workout includes

- a pushing exercise (a press or a push-up)
- a pulling exercise (a row or pulldown)

- a deadlift or squat variation (because these are the heaviest and most exhausting movements in the program, you'll do one in Workout A and the other in Workout B of each stage)
- a single-leg or split-stance exercise (such as a lunge or step-up variation)

Your goal, within each stage, is to improve your performance in every strength exercise from one workout to the next, culminating in a peak of sorts in the final workouts of that stage. Then you move on to the next stage, with new exercises and new combinations of sets and reps.

INTERVAL TRAINING

Interval training involves drills in which you go as hard as you can for a designated amount of time, recover, and then go again. Alwyn changes the exact parameters as you go along, but the idea is the same: Improve from one workout to the next, just as you do in the strength exercises. The goal is to have your best performance in the final workouts of each stage. Then you move on to the next set of challenges.

You have a wide range of choices for how you do the intervals, as you'll learn in the next chapter. (Some specific exercises are shown and described in Chapter 15.) Most of you, most of the time, will probably do them indoors, where your choices include cardio machines (like a treadmill or stationary bike), a sled (which you can push or pull), or strength equipment (which you use for carries). Or you can go outdoors and do intervals on a road or track or in a park.

Most workouts will take 50 to 60 minutes. In each stage, the first workouts will be shorter; they'll get longer as you add intervals and take more recovery time between sets. If you finish in less time, you're probably working too fast, and at too low an intensity level, to get the benefits of a serious training program. If they take longer than 60 minutes, and that's an issue for you, you can break the workouts up by doing the intervals on separate days.

EXERCISE SELECTION

One of the first questions you'll have, when you look at the workouts in the next three chapters, is whether you can substitute exercises. Sometimes you'll need to make adjustments because of the space or equipment you have. Other times you'll find that your body doesn't like the designated exercise, and you'll wonder if it's okay to take a step back to an earlier version of the same movement pattern or jump ahead to one that's slightly more advanced.

We encourage you to make adjustments to fit your equipment, circumstances, and goals, as long as you stay within the category. So you can substitute one squat variation for another, or a press for a press. A few guidelines:

- Never do an exercise that hurts. If one bench press variation hurts your shoulder or a lunge variation hurts your knee, swap it out for one that allows you a pain-free range of motion.
- It's okay to stick with one variation for multiple stages if you like the exercise, you're getting stronger every workout, and you don't feel you're ready for more advanced exercises within that movement pattern. This is especially true for squats. We start everyone with the goblet squat, a great exercise that was developed by our friend Dan John. A novice lifter could use it for months and still see progress.
- It's also okay to jump ahead if the prescribed variation is too easy for you. We recommend that you at least try each one, but if you easily get all the sets and reps and don't feel challenged, go ahead and try the next one.
- All of us are limited by our equipment. If you don't have kettlebells, a suspension system, sliding discs, or a sled, you can't do the variations that require those tools.

EQUIPMENT REQUIREMENTS AND OPTIONS

If you've never done a serious training program and aren't familiar with these basic tools, please go to Appendix B for a complete explanation of each and tips on how to how to acquire it for a home gym without dipping into your retirement account.

Here's what you need for the workouts in *Strong*:

- Dumbbells (you'll need a range of weights)
- Barbell and plates (preferably an Olympic barbell)
- Chin-up bar
- A power rack, squat stands, or some other way to elevate a barbell for squats, inverted rows, and other exercises
- A cable machine *or* a range of resistance bands and tubing
- A bench (preferably one that inclines)

- A sturdy box or step
- A clock or timer

Here's what you'll probably want, sooner or later:

- Kettlebells
- A suspension trainer (like the TRX) and/or a Swiss ball for exercises that call for an unstable base
- Bands or tubing (even if you have access to a cable machine)
- A foam roller
- Valslides, or a similar type of disc that slides across carpets or wood floors
- Heart-rate monitor (for the intervals, starting in Stage 3)

HOW TO BE AWESOME

With apologies for repeating something we covered earlier: *Your effort is the key to success* in this or any other training program. The best program in the world won't give you results you haven't earned. And, as any good trainer knows, even a crappy program will give you results if you push yourself hard enough. But the real magic happens when you apply great effort to a great program like Alwyn's.

These habits and practices ensure the best possible results:

Always log your workouts. Most of the benefits of Alwyn's program come from improving your performance in the strength exercises. Improvement isn't *just* about numbers; it's hard to quantify knowledge and skill, both of which are invaluable. But the numbers are the most reliable way to gauge your progress in a training program. Your training log is your score sheet. If it's not there, you didn't do it. If it is there, you know exactly where you started, how far you've come, and most important, what you need to do next.

How you track your workouts is up to you.

We have free downloadable training logs available at werkit.com, showing each workout on a single page. Or you can simply photocopy the workout charts on the following pages if you have the paper version of the book. If you have an ebook, you should be able to open it on a computer screen and then print the charts from each page. (Sometimes it's easier to make a screen capture and then print that, rather than trying to print the page directly.)

Personally, I just write everything down in a spiral notebook. It takes seconds, and it's easy to flip back a page or two to see what I've done in previous workouts, and thus what I need to do in the current one.

I admit I'm a bit of a techno-skeptic, but that's not the only reason I prefer the old paper-and-pen approach. The simplicity of it allows me to stay focused on the workout. It also lets me control the pace of my own training. I don't want my recovery between sets dictated by how long it takes to record my results.

A no-tech log also gives you a complete break from both home and work. Almost all our work involves a computer screen, and much of family life is coordinated through texts and phone calls. A workout might be the only freedom you get from constant connectivity with customers, coworkers, bosses, friends, and family members. Why bring that technology into the weight room if you don't have to?

That said, I know a lot of readers prefer high-tech to low. I'm in favor of whatever works for you.

Make each workout matter. In each stage, as you know, you'll be using new exercises and different combinations of sets and reps. That means your first workouts in each stage—the first time you do Workout A and Workout B—will involve two different processes:

- Learning the exercises
- Figuring out appropriate weights

If you've done this before, you know the latter process involves trial and error, especially when learning new or unfamiliar exercises. (If you *haven't* done it before, and have no idea how to select appropriate weights, please see Appendix C, "How Much Weight Should I Use?") Don't worry about getting it exactly right. You're just trying to set a baseline. As long as the workout still feels like a workout, you've done it right.

The goal of each subsequent workout, as you also know, is to improve upon that baseline, either by using heavier weights or by completing more repetitions with the original weight.

Be the voice of reason. Two questions that come up a lot:

Should I work out when I feel sick?
How do I train around this injury I have?

I admire the motivation it takes to ask the questions. You probably train harder than almost anyone you know and feel like every missed workout is a lost opportunity to improve. But sometimes not working out is the best use of your workout time.

Training is a form of stress, one you impose on your body with the goal of getting better at something that matters to you. When the goal is strength, you create levels of tension that challenge your muscles to get bigger and stronger. No stress means no results. But too much stress can be even worse, leaving you with an injury, excessive soreness, or fatigue that requires so much recovery time you lose some of the strength and muscle quality you already have.

Illness is also a form of stress, one that challenges your body to become resilient to whatever pathogen made you sick. Common sense tells you that adding another type of stress will overload your immune system, make the original illness worse, and require more recovery time, once again causing you to lose some of your strength.

Granted, you'll quickly regain what you lost, once you've recovered and you're back to training without limitations. But it's still a setback—an unforced error that could easily have been avoided if you'd listened to that voice in your head.

When I asked Alwyn the injury question, his response was unequivocal: "I really don't like the idea of working around an actual injury so you can do heavy strength work." It came up because of a comment from a reader, who suggested that our next book include specific tips for someone who has a torn rotator cuff, sciatica, and chronic lower-back pain from a herniated disc. "That's not a training book," Alwyn said. "That's an ER appointment!"

Don't look for ways to work around a serious, acute injury. Fix it if it can be fixed, preferably with the guidance of a doctor or physical therapist. If it can't be fixed, or if the surgical repair might create problems of its own, then you have to make tough choices.

But always start with the most obvious one: Don't do anything to make it worse.

7

Phase One: Develop

I LEARNED EARLY IN MY FITNESS-WRITING career that there's no such thing as a beginner. Originally I thought it was a guy thing. You know, just as every 16-year-old boy wants to change his last name to Earnhardt the day he gets his driver's license, so every adult male who picks up a dumbbell imagines that he's Arnold Schwarzenegger's secret love child. No matter how average we appear, we all believe there's a Comstock Lode of awesomeness deep inside, just waiting to be revealed.

Lesson learned: Always assume a male reader regards himself as more advanced than he is and then try to convince him to begin a program at the beginning despite his inclination to go straight to the middle.

We published *NROL for Women* assuming the opposite: that young, healthy women with years of fitness experience held themselves back by doing beginner workouts in perpetuity. So our goal was to convince women to push themselves to the middle.

Now Alwyn and I face an interesting quandary: Many of you reading this really *are* intermediate lifters, if not advanced. And you have the exact same question we heard thousands of times from guys: "Since I'm not a beginner, why should I start at the beginning?"

Alwyn, as you'd expect, has given it some thought. "I'm a fourth-degree black belt in tae kwon do," he told me. "I've been a black belt for 27 years now, way more than half my life. But if I started Shotokan karate tomorrow, I'd be a white belt, because that's where everyone starts."

If you can't relate to a martial arts analogy, Alwyn has one we can all understand. The best runners in the world begin each race from the exact same spot: the starting line. The champions get to the finish line a lot faster than the others, but they don't get to start any closer to it. And if one of those champion runners happened to show up at Results Fitness to train with Alwyn, he'd start them off exactly where he starts you: with workouts pretty close to those in Stage 1.

Now, much as I'd like to think you've been persuaded by our masterful arguments, I've circled this drain enough times to know many of you haven't. So let's get extremely specific, beginning with the readers who *absolutely* need to start here:

- If you're an entry-level lifter, or if your training experience is limited to machines at your health club, random exercises from websites, or DVDs with "10 minutes" in the title, you're a beginner.
- If you've never done a structured program, no matter how long you've been working out, you aren't *literally* a beginner, but you're still at the front end of the learning curve.
- Same goes for someone who works out but hasn't learned the key strength exercises, like squats, deadlifts, presses, and rows using a barbell or dumbbells.
- Finally, if you're familiar with the major exercises but haven't done one of Alwyn's NROL programs, you *really* don't want to start in the middle. You won't have the foundation you need for the more intense workouts of Phase Two and Phase Three.

For everyone else, here's why I hope you'll start with Phase One, even though you may not want to:

- If you did the programs in *NROL for Women* but not in subsequent NROL books, you'll find these very different. You need some time to get the hang of them.

- If you did one or more of those programs in the past, but moved on after you completed them, you're best served by starting here. You may be surprised to find that some of the exercises and techniques you once mastered didn't stay mastered. You'll get it back faster than you acquired it, and you'll be happy you did.
- Even if you just completed the *Supercharged* program last week, you may have already lost some of the fitness qualities you developed in the earliest workouts.

Finally, *if your body has changed* since the last time you did an introductory workout (injury, childbirth, menopause, significant weight gain or loss), or your circumstances are different (more stressful job or home situation, erratic training schedule, poor sleep), it's a good idea to go back to the beginning and start over. Your brain remembers what you could do before the change, but your body doesn't.

I can't speak from experience about childbirth or menopause. But I know a few things about getting older. (And learn more every year, alas.) I know the frustration of diminished abilities. I know how it feels to have a body that can't do what it could even five years ago. I also know the benefits of circling back to the starting line, which rise exponentially when compared to the downside of jumping ahead to advanced workouts when your body isn't ready. The risk is high even when your body *is* ready. You don't know where the wall is until you run into it, and injuries like to lurk in the shadows of ambition.

So that's our pitch for all of you to start with Phase One. If you're still with me, let's get into it.

HOW TO READ THE WORKOUT CHARTS

If this is your first rodeo with Alwyn's programs, here's a quick guide to the structure and terminology.

1a, 1b, Etc.

When you see a number and letter in front of an exercise, it indicates *alternating sets*. Do the first exercise (1a), and rest. Then do the second exercise (1b), and rest. Continue alternating until you finish all the sets of those exercises, with rest in between. Then move on to the next pair of exercises.

STAGE 1

Workout A

Exercise	Sets × Reps	Workout 1	Workout 2	Workout 3	Workout 4
Core					
1a. Plank	1–2 × 60 seconds				
1b. Bird dog	4 × 15 seconds*				
Strength					
2a. Goblet squat	2 × 12				
2b. Dumbbell 3-point row	2 × 12*				
3a. Step-up	2 × 12*				
3b. Push-up	2 × 12				
Intervals					
	3–6 × 60 seconds work/ 120 seconds rest†				

Suggested rest time between sets: up to 60 seconds.

* Each side.

† See instructions on p. 57.

STAGE 1

Workout B

Exercise	Sets × Reps	Workout 1	Workout 2	Workout 3	Workout 4
Core					
1a. Side plank	1–2 × 30 seconds*				
1b. Cable half-kneeling antirotation press	1–2 × 3*†				
Strength					
2a. Single-leg Romanian deadlift with reach	2 × 12*				
2b. Push-up variation‡	2 × 12				
3a. Split squat	2 × 12*				
3b. Inverted row	2 × 12				
Intervals					
	3–6 × 60 seconds work/120 seconds rest§				

Suggested rest time between sets: up to 60 seconds.

* Each side.

† Hold each press for 10 seconds; a set is 30 seconds per side.

‡ Alwyn recommends the suspended chest press for this workout. But if you don't have access to a suspension system (like the TRX), you can do any push-up variation shown in Chapter 14, as long as it's different from the one you selected for Workout A.

§ See instructions on p. 57.

If you see more than two exercises grouped together (2a, 2b, 2c, and 2d, for example), you do it the exact same way, finishing all four exercises in order before repeating them.

When you see a number without a letter, do that exercise as *straight sets*. Do the first set, rest, and continue until you finish.

"Do I *Have* to Alternate Exercises?"

Sometimes your gym is too crowded, and you can't tie up more than one station at a time. Or you're working out at home with limited equipment, and it takes too much time to change weights. Or, for whatever reason, you just prefer to focus on one exercise at a time.

Do what you have to do. I don't know of any research showing that alternating sets are better than straight sets for any important goal.

That said, Alwyn prefers alternating sets because they allow more recovery between each set of an exercise. For example, if you do a set of squats, rest 60 seconds, and repeat, you obviously have 60 seconds of recovery time. But let's say you're alternating squats with dumbbell rows. You do a set of squats, rest 60 seconds, then do a set of rows with each arm, which takes 60 seconds. Then you rest another 60 seconds. Now your lower-body muscles have 180 seconds of recovery before your second set of squats—three times as much as they'd get with straight sets. The extra time means you'll be able to use a heavier weight and probably get a couple more reps with it. You've also used your time efficiently by doing an upper-body exercise while recovering.

"Can I Do More Than 2 Sets Per Exercise?"

Kind of. What Alwyn wants you to do here is push yourself really hard on those 2 sets, and improve your performance each time. But that's a challenge when you aren't sure how much weight to use on your first set. My solution, when I did these workouts, was to add a warm-up set to some or all of the strength exercises.

Start with a weight you're pretty sure isn't enough to exhaust your muscles after 12 reps. Do 10 reps with it. Then increase the weight, and shoot for 12 on your 2 work sets.

It's probably not practical to do warm-up sets for the body-weight exercises, like the inverted row in Workout B and the push-up variations in both A and B. I suppose you could do easier versions for a warm-up set, but in my own workouts I didn't find it necessary.

Recovery Time

As you can see from our phrasing, "suggested rest time between sets" is a guideline, not a rule. The goal is to encourage you to slow down, use heavier weights, and push yourself hard enough on each set that you need some recovery time. Maybe 60 seconds is more than you need in Stage 1, but as you get deeper into the program, you'll find yourself using every bit of it.

"Do I Rest Between Arms on the Rows or Between Legs on the Step-Ups?"

Depends. In these Phase One workouts, it's best to do all your reps with one arm or leg (you probably want to start with your nondominant limb—your left if you're right-handed), then switch positions and immediately repeat with the other side. But if you feel like you need a break between limbs, take one. You don't want to do 12 reps when you're gasping for breath before the first one. The stronger you get, the more likely you are to work with a weight heavy enough to leave you gassed after working one limb.

Workout 1, Workout 2, Etc.

Workout 1 is the first time you do that workout. Workout 2 is the second time. Here's how it looks over four weeks:

	Monday	Tuesday	Wednesday	Thursday	Friday	Saturday	Sunday
Week 1	A: Workout 1	off	B: Workout 1	off	A: Workout 2	off	off
Week 2	B: Workout 2	off	A: Workout 3	off	B: Workout 3	off	off
Week 3	A: Workout 4	off	B: Workout 4	off	A: Workout 5	off	off
Week 4	B: Workout 5	off	A: Workout 6	off	B: Workout 6	off	off

Use those columns on your training log to record your results on each set. You'll notice that the log stops at Workout 4, even though many of you will do each workout six times, as shown in this grid. There's a very sophisticated reason: It's all we could fit on the page. (I apologize for the technical jargon.) So you'll need to make two copies of each training log to record six workouts.

Intervals

Veterans of *NROL for Women* will recognize Alwyn's format: 1 minute of work, followed by 2 minutes of recovery. For others, it may run counter to your idea of what intervals should be. The most common is 30 seconds of work—just long enough to get out of breath—followed by 60 seconds of recovery, with the goal of reducing your recovery time until the ratio of work to rest is one to one.

These are different; 60 seconds is a *long* time to go at a furious pace. But if you don't work yourself into a lather, those 2 minutes of recovery will feel interminable. Worst-case scenario, you end up doing a few minutes of aerobics, going a little harder for a minute and a little easier for the next two.

That's why Alwyn has you start off with just three intervals. You have no reason to hold anything back.

HOW IT WORKS

Let's look at the simplest option for interval work, a stationary bike at your gym.

Time	Tension Level	Pace
0:00–0:30	1 or 2	80–90 rpm
0:30–1:30	4 to 6	110–120 rpm
1:30–3:30	1 or 2	80–90 rpm
3:30–4:30	5 or 6	110–120 rpm
4:30–6:30	1 or 2	80–90 rpm
6:30–7:30	5 or 6	110–120 rpm
7:30–8:00	1 or 2	80–90 rpm

The suggested tension levels are just an example. All bikes are different. I have a spin bike at my gym, so I have to crank the tension all the way up to 10 or 11 to make it challenging enough. You have three chances to get it right in your first workout. Once you get the right tension for both work and recovery, you probably want to keep it at those levels for subsequent workouts as you add an interval each time. You're making progress with volume—the total amount of work you do—rather than intensity. (That said, if you can also increase the tension, without sacrificing volume, that's even better.)

ADDING INTERVALS

There are two different progressions for adding intervals:

1. **If You're Doing Workout A and Workout B Six Times Each, Add One Interval a Week**
   Let's say you're lifting three times a week. In the first week, you'll do three intervals after each workout: Workout A on Monday, Workout B on Wednesday, and Workout A again on Friday. The next week, you'll do four. You'll do five the third week, then six in the fourth and final week of Stage 1.

2. **If You're Doing Workout A and Workout B Four Times Each, Add One Interval Each Time You Repeat the Workout**
   The first time you do Workout A and Workout B—Monday and Wednesday—you'll do three intervals. The next time—Friday and Monday of the following week—you'll do four. Then five the third time, and six the fourth and final time.

"Do I Use the Same Equipment Each Time?"

I wouldn't, if you can avoid it. It will get old fast. If you're lifting three times a week, and doing Workout A and Workout B six times each, I recommend using three different machines or sets of exercises. If you use a stationary bike on Monday, you might use a rowing machine on Wednesday and an elliptical machine on Friday. Just make sure you use those machines on the same days throughout Stage 1: stationary bike Monday, rowing machine Wednesday, elliptical machine Friday. That way you know you're making progress from week to week.

If you're among the more advanced readers and doing Workout A and Workout B just four times each, use one for A and another for B. You have a world of options beyond cardio machines:

- Pushing or pulling a sled
- Jumping rope
- Battling ropes
- Kettlebell swings
- Punching or kicking a heavy bag
- Loaded carries (shown in Chapter 15)

If it's something you can sustain for a minute, and then repeat several more times, you can use it.

Special Workout

Do this workout one time, after completing Stage 1. On all exercises, use the same weights as Workout 2. If you did advanced variations of the body-weight exercises—planks, side planks, push-ups, inverted rows—try to replicate the ones you used the second time you did each workout.

Exercise	Sets × Reps	Results
Core		
1a. Plank	1 × ALAP	
1b. Side plank	1 × ALAP*	
Strength		
2a. Goblet squat	1 × AMRAP	
2b. Dumbbell 3-point row	1 × AMRAP*	
3a. Push-up	1 × AMRAP	
3b. Split squat	1 × AMRAP*	
3c. Inverted row	1 × AMRAP	

ALAP = as long as possible; *AMRAP* = as many reps as possible.

Suggested rest time between sets: 60 seconds.

* Each side.

STAGE 2

Workout A

Exercise	Sets × Reps	Workout 1	Workout 2	Workout 3	Workout 4
Core					
1. Plank with pulldown	1–2 × 12*				
Strength					
2a. Reverse lunge	2–3 × 10*				
2b. Inverted row	2–3 × 10				
3a. Romanian deadlift	2–3 × 10				
3b. Push-up	2–3 × 10				
Intervals					
	5–8 × 60 seconds work/90 seconds rest†				

Suggested rest time between sets: up to 60 seconds.

* Each side.

† Start with 5, and add intervals as described for Stage 1.

STAGE 2

Workout B

Exercise	Sets × Reps	Workout 1	Workout 2	Workout 3	Workout 4
Core					
1. Side plank with row	1–2 × 12*				
Strength					
2a. Suspended lunge and touch†	2–3 × 10*				
2b. Dumbbell bench press	2–3 × 10				
3a. Front squat	2–3 × 10				
3b. Standing single-arm cable row	2–3 × 10*				
Intervals					
	5–8 × 60 seconds work/90 seconds rest‡				

Suggested rest time between sets: up to 60 seconds.

* Each side.

† If you don't have access to a suspension system, you can do the single-leg Romanian deadlift instead.

‡ Start with 5, and add intervals as described for Stage 1.

STAGE 3

Workout A

Exercise	Sets × Reps	Workout 1	Workout 2	Workout 3	Workout 4
Core					
1. Valslide push-away	1–2 × 12*				
Strength					
2a. Single-arm deadlift	3 × 8†				
2b. Dumbbell incline bench press	3 × 8				
2c. Rear-foot-elevated split squat	3 × 8‡				
2d. Half-kneeling X pulldown	3 × 8				
Intervals					
	AMRAP × 60 seconds work/heart rate recovery in 10 minutes§				

AMRAP = as many reps as possible.

Suggested rest time between sets: up to 60 seconds.

* This means 12 total reps, 6 with each arm. If you don't have Valslides or the equivalent, you'll find alternatives in Appendix B.

† This means 8 total reps. Alwyn recommends alternating arms each set. So you might do 8 with your right arm on the first set, 8 with your left on the second, and 4 with each arm in the third, switching halfway through the set.

‡ Each side.

§ For explanation, see p. 62.

STAGE 3

Workout B

Exercise	Sets × Reps	Workout 1	Workout 2	Workout 3	Workout 4
Core					
1. Alternating side plank	1–2 × 5*†				
Strength					
2a. Back squat with pause	3 × 8				
2b. Dumbbell single-arm dead-stop row	3 × 8*				
2c. Single-leg Romanian deadlift from box	3 × 8*				
2d. Suspended push-up	3 × 8				
Intervals					
	AMRAP × 60 seconds work/heart rate recovery in 10 minutes‡				

AMRAP = as many reps as possible.

Suggested rest time between sets: up to 60 seconds.

* Each side.

† Hold each side plank for 3 seconds; should take 45–50 seconds total.

‡ For explanation, see below.

INTERVALS WITH HEART-RATE RECOVERY

In a 1-minute interval, your heart rate should rise to 80 to 90 percent of your maximum heart rate (MHR). The more fit you are, the faster your heart rate will recover. You want to begin the next interval as soon it falls to 65 percent of your max. That might happen in 45 seconds after the first interval, but take 60 seconds or more after the fifth or sixth.

You want to do as many intervals as you can in 10 minutes, with the goal of completing more as your conditioning improves.

Here's how it works:

If You Have a Heart-Rate Monitor

Step 1. Estimate your MHR by subtracting your age from 220. If you're 30, 220 − 30 = 190 beats per minute (bpm).

Step 2. Calculate 65 percent of your MHR to get your recovery heart rate. In this example, $190 \times 0.65 = 123$ bpm.

Step 3. Set your heart-rate monitor to beep when your heart rate reaches 123. That's your signal to begin the next interval.

If You Don't Have a Heart-Rate Monitor

Without a monitor, you can check your own pulse for 10 seconds to get a (very rough) estimate of your heart rate. Use the same formula to determine your MHR and 65 percent of your max. Now divide by 6. In this example, $123 \div 6 = 20.5$. When you reach 20 or 21 beats in 10 seconds, you're ready to start the next interval.

Or you can make it much simpler, and start the next interval when your breathing returns to normal and you feel you're ready to go.

8

Phase Two: Demand

In Phase One Alwyn gave you three ways to make progress.

1. Load
   You use a little more weight each time you repeat a workout within a stage. And you use lower reps from one stage to the next, which by definition means heavier weights.
2. Volume
   You do a little more total work, increasing from 1 or 2 sets per exercise to 3 sets. (That's in addition to the volume you add in the intervals.)
3. Exercise selection
   Alwyn took you from basic exercises in each movement pattern to more advanced variations: goblet squats to front squats to paused back squats, for example.

All three are examples of *linear periodization*, a simple, straightforward way to make incremental improvements toward a larger goal: to get leaner, stronger, and more skilled. Now you're going to do the same, only faster, using *undulating periodization*.

As before, you have two workouts—A and B—in each phase. But you're going to do each of those workouts with three different configurations of sets and reps, while using the same exercises. You'll change the weights you use accordingly: a little more weight when you do lower reps, a little less for higher reps. Since your goal of making each workout matter remains the same, you want to improve your performance within each of those three rep ranges. So if you use X the first time you do 3 sets of 10 reps, you want to use X + *something* the next time.

That's the undulating part, and it's a lot to keep track of. If you didn't use training logs in Phase One, you sure as hell need them now.

Meanwhile, you're still using elements of classic periodization. The average number of reps you do per exercise in Phase Two decreases as you work through Stages 4, 5, and 6. That means you'll use increasingly heavier weights over the next three months. Using heavier weights automatically makes the exercises themselves more demanding. Low-rep sets with near-maximal weights will take a lot more out of you than the same exercise done with lighter weights for double-digit reps.

A QUICK GUIDE TO THE WORKOUT CHARTS

In Phase One, you had just two workout charts per stage—one for Workout A, one for Workout B. Now you'll have three for Workout A, one for each configuration of sets and reps, and another three for Workout B. That's six per stage. A month of training will look like this for Stage 4:

	Monday	Tuesday	Wednesday	Thursday	Friday	Saturday	Sunday
Week 1	A: Workout 1 (2 × 15)	off	B: Workout 1 (3 × 12)	off	A: Workout 2 (3 × 10)	off	off
Week 2	B: Workout 2 (2 × 15)	off	A: Workout 3 (3 × 12)	off	B: Workout 3 (3 × 10)	off	off
Week 3	A: Workout 4 (2 × 15)	off	B: Workout 4 (3 × 12)	off	A: Workout 5⇨ (3 × 10)	off	off
Week 4	B: Workout 5 (2 × 15)	off	A: Workout 6 (3 × 12)	off	B: Workout 6⇨ (3 × 10)	off	off

With a glance you get the basic ideas:

• You'll do 2 sets of 15 reps each Monday (or whenever you do the first workout of the week), 3 sets of 12 on Wednesday, and 3 sets of 10 on Friday.

- It takes two weeks to do all three configurations of the A and B workouts.
- The second two weeks repeat the first two weeks, only with heavier weights on all the strength exercises.

(See "Repping Out" on p. 68 for an explanation of the ⇨ symbol.)

INTERVALS IN PHASE TWO

Alwyn started Phase One with a very simple interval-training method: *fixed work, fixed recovery.* In Stage 1 you worked hard for 60 seconds and recovered for 120 seconds. The ratio of work to recovery, in equation form, was 1:2. In Stage 2, it shifted to 60 seconds of work with 90 seconds of recovery, or a ratio of 1:1.5.

He then introduced a new method in Stage 3: *fixed work, variable recovery.* Your work interval was still 60 seconds, but you monitored your heart rate to determine when it was time to begin the next bout. (Without a heart-rate monitor, you checked your pulse or waited until your breathing returned to normal before starting the next interval.)

Throughout Phase Two you'll employ Alwyn's preferred method, the one he believes is by far the best way to do intervals: *variable work, variable recovery.* Work until you reach 85 percent of your MHR (see p. 62). Then go easy until you drop to 65 percent of your MHR. Set your heart-rate monitor to beep at 85 and 65 percent, and you're all set. Do that for 10 minutes at the end of each workout, with the goal of increasing your performance—the number of intervals completed—each week.

"What If I Don't Have a Heart-Rate Monitor?"

In that case, stick with *fixed work, variable recovery.* Lower your work interval to 45 seconds, and begin the next one when you've reached full recovery, determined by either monitoring your pulse for 10 seconds or when your breath returns to normal.

"Should I Do the Same Thing Each Workout?"

You can, but I don't recommend it. I think you'll get the best results, and the most enjoyment (or the least boredom), from picking three different options, one for each workout in a typical week. Just make sure you do the same things from week to week. So if you use a rowing machine on Monday, use the same machine the following Monday. If there's too much variety, then you aren't really training anything. It's just a random collection of short, challenging episodes.

Now, if that's what you *prefer*, never mind what I just said. Just as doing something is almost always better than doing nothing, doing something you like is almost always better than doing something you hate or you find tedious and uninspiring.

I also recommend mixing it up for each stage. Try different combinations of machines and other exercises. In the previous chapter I gave you a list of options you might find in a well-equipped gym: sled (for pushing and pulling), jump rope, battling ropes, kettlebells (for swings and carries), heavy bag (for punching and kicking).

You can use one of those options for a 10-minute session or you can combine them in a circuit. Let's say your gym has an open space for sleds, carries, and other locomotion exercises. You could do a circuit like this:

- Sled push to 85 percent of MHR
- Recover to 65 percent of MHR
- Overhead carry (with kettlebells, dumbbells, or a barbell) to 85 percent of MHR
- Recover to 65 percent of MHR
- Sled pull to 85 percent of MHR
- Recover to 65 percent of MHR
- Farmer's walk (with kettlebells or dumbbells held at your sides) to 85 percent of MHR
- Recover to 65 percent of MHR

And then repeat the sequence.

"So Intervals Are Always 10 Minutes?"

Yes.

"Does the Final Recovery Count Toward the 10 Minutes?"

It doesn't have to. If you push hard to hit 85 percent of MHR right at the 10-minute mark, you can take as much or as little time as you want to recover. If I'm on a stationary bike I'll usually slow down for 30 seconds after the last bout just because it's what my legs want to do. It's probably the same on a treadmill.

But if I'm pushing a sled or carrying something heavy, I'm happy to stop once I've completed the interval. Just putting the equipment away feels like more work than I should have to do.

REPPING OUT

In Workout A5 and Workout B6, you'll see an arrow symbol (⇨). That's your signal to *rep out* on the final set, doing as many repetitions as you can. You might not be able to do more than 10, in which case you can congratulate yourself for choosing exactly the right weight. You might do 12 or 13, in which case you can congratulate yourself for being such a badass that you blew right past what you thought was your 10-rep max. Or you might not even get to 10, in which case you should congratulate yourself for being so ambitious with your weight selection.

Repping out is the equivalent of the Special Workout at the end of Phase 1. For that one set, you don't stop until you reach complete muscular exhaustion and can't do another rep with good form.

RECOVERY BETWEEN SETS, CORE TRAINING, AND WORKOUT LENGTH

Observant readers will notice that the suggested rest time between sets now varies according to the rep range, with longer recovery for lower reps per set. You'll also see more core exercises, some of which require setup time. If you train in a health club, you may need to do them in different areas. Even if you have the weight room to yourself, or have a home gym so well equipped that Mark Wahlberg is jealous, these workouts take more time than those in Phase One.

Many readers over the years have told me that workouts beyond a certain length are inconvenient for them, if not impossible. So if these workouts go past your limit, you have a couple of options. The most obvious is to do the intervals on separate days. Alwyn prefers that you don't; there's something about the combination of exhausting resistance training and exhausting intervals that works better for body composition than either by itself. (*Why* it works better is still something of a mystery.) But as the man said, the perfect is the enemy of the good, and we all have to do what we can, when we can.

The second option is slightly worse: Do the core exercises *and* the intervals on separate days. That should reduce the workout to 45 minutes, at most.

STAGE 4

Workout A: 1 and 4

Exercise	Sets × Reps	Workout 1	Workout 4
Core			
1a. Suspended plank	1–2 × 60 seconds		
1b. Bird dog	4 × 15 seconds*†		
2. Half-kneeling cable chop	2 × 10*		
Strength			
3a. Back squat	2 × 15		
3b. Chin-up, band-assisted chin-up, or lat pulldown	2 × 15		
4a. Step-up	2 × 15*		
4b. Dumbbell bench press	2 × 15		
Intervals			
	AMRAP × 85% MHR/65% MHR in 10 minutes‡		

AMRAP = as many reps as possible; *MHR* = maximum heart rate.

Suggested rest time between sets: up to 60 seconds.

* Each side.

† You can do this twice, alternating with the plank. Or you can do a single set of bird dogs in between sets of the plank. Or you can do a single set of each.

‡ For explanation, see p. 66.

STAGE 4

Workout A: 2 and 5

Exercise	Sets × Reps	Workout 2	Workout 5 ⇨
Core			
1a. Suspended plank	1–2 × 60 seconds		
1b. Bird dog	4 × 15 seconds*†		
2. Half-kneeling cable chop	2 × 10*		
Strength			
3a. Back squat	3 × 10		
3b. Chin-up, band-assisted chin-up, or lat pulldown	3 × 10		
4a. Step-up	3 × 10*		
4b. Dumbbell bench press	3 × 10		
Intervals			
	AMRAP × 85% MHR/65% MHR in 10 minutes‡		

AMRAP = as many reps as possible; *MHR* = maximum heart rate; ⇨ = rep out on final set of each strength exercise in Workout 5.

Suggested rest time between sets: 60 seconds.

* Each side.

† You can do this twice, alternating with the plank. Or you can do a single set of bird dogs in between sets of the plank. Or you can do a single set of each.

‡ For explanation, see p. 66.

STAGE 4

Workout A: 3 and 6

Exercise	Sets × Reps	Workout 3	Workout 6
Core			
1a. Suspended plank	1–2 × 60 seconds		
1b. Bird dog	4 × 15 seconds*†		
2. Half-kneeling cable chop	2 × 10*		
Strength			
3a. Back squat	3 × 12		
3b. Chin-up, band-assisted chin-up, or lat pulldown	3 × 12		
4a. Step-up	3 × 12*		
4b. Dumbbell bench press	3 × 12		
Intervals			
	AMRAP × 85% MHR/65% MHR in 10 minutes‡		

AMRAP = as many reps as possible; *MHR* = maximum heart rate.

Suggested rest time between sets: up to 60 seconds.

* Each side.

† You can do this twice, alternating with the plank. Or you can do a single set of bird dogs in between sets of the plank. Or you can do a single set of each.

‡ For explanation, see p. 66.

STAGE 4

Workout B: 1 and 4

Exercise	Sets × Reps	Workout 1	Workout 4
Core			
1. Suspended side plank	1–2 x 60 seconds*		
2. Half-kneeling cable lift	2 × 10*		
Strength			
3a. Deadlift from blocks	3 × 12		
3b. Push-up variation†	3 × 12		
4a. Side lunge and touch	3 × 12*		
4b. Standing single-arm low-cable row	3 × 12*		
Intervals			
	AMRAP × 85% MHR/65% MHR in 10 minutes‡		

AMRAP = as many reps as possible; *MHR* = maximum heart rate.

Suggested rest time between sets: up to 60 seconds.

* Each side.

† Use a different variation for each rep range.

‡ For explanation, see p. 66.

STAGE 4

Workout B: 2 and 5

Exercise	Sets × Reps	Workout 2	Workout 5
Core			
1. Suspended side plank	1–2 × 60 seconds*		
2. Half-kneeling cable lift	2 × 10*		
Strength			
3a. Deadlift from blocks	2 × 15		
3b. Push-up variation[†]	2 × 15		
4a. Side lunge and touch	2 × 15*		
4b. Standing single-arm low-cable row	2 × 15*		
Intervals			
	AMRAP × 85% MHR/65% MHR in 10 minutes[‡]		

AMRAP = as many reps as possible; *MHR* = maximum heart rate.

Suggested rest time between sets: up to 60 seconds.

* Each side.

[†] Use a different variation for each rep range.

[‡] For explanation, see p. 66.

STAGE 4

Workout B: 3 and 6

Exercise	Sets × Reps	Workout 3	Workout 6 ⇨
Core			
1. Suspended side plank	1–2 × 60 seconds*		
2. Half-kneeling cable lift	2 × 10*		
Strength			
3a. Deadlift from blocks	3 × 10		
3b. Push-up variation[†]	3 × 10		
4a. Side lunge and touch	3 × 10*		
4b. Standing single-arm low-cable row	3 × 10*		
Intervals			
	AMRAP × 85% MHR/65% MHR in 10 minutes[‡]		

AMRAP = as many reps as possible; MHR = maximum heart rate; ⇨ = rep out on final set of each strength exercise in Workout 6.

Suggested rest time between sets: 60 seconds.

* Each side.

[†] Use a different variation for each rep range.

[‡] For explanation, see p. 66.

STAGE 5

Here's what a month of training will look like:

	Monday	Tuesday	Wednesday	Thursday	Friday	Saturday	Sunday
Week 1	A: Workout 1 (2–3 × 12)	off	B: Workout 1 (2–3 × 10)	off	A: Workout 2 (3–4 × 8)	off	off
Week 2	B: Workout 2 (2–3 × 12)	off	A: Workout 3 (2–3 × 10)	off	B: Workout 3 (3–4 × 8)	off	off
Week 3	A: Workout 4 (2–3 × 12)	off	B: Workout 4 (2–3 × 10)	off	A: Workout 5 ⇨ (3–4 × 8)	off	off
Week 4	B: Workout 5 (2–3 × 12)	off	A: Workout 6 (2–3 × 10)	off	B: Workout 6 ⇨ (3–4 × 8)	off	off

"Why 2–3 or 3–4 Sets? Why Don't You Pick One?"

If you want to keep it simple, do this:

- If the workout calls for 2 or 3 sets, do 2 sets in the first half of the stage (your first time through each rep range) and 3 sets in the final workouts.
- If the workout calls for 3 or 4 sets, do 3 in the first half of the stage, and 4 in the second half.

There's also a nonsimple answer. You can make decisions on the spot, based on how the workout is going and what you think you can and should do. Trainers call this *autoregulation*. The better you know your body, the better you can autoregulate each workout without compromising its benefits.

The ultimate goal of each workout is to do something better than in the previous one. That can include

- Using a heavier weight
- Doing more reps with the previous weight
- Doing more total volume (sets + reps) with the previous weight

What you're looking for is that moment when you say to yourself, "Nailed it!" If you can say that after 2 or 3 sets, you may decide not to do the third or fourth. If not, then you probably need that final set to make the workout a success.

STAGE 5

Workout A: 1 and 4

Exercise	Sets × Reps	Workout 1	Workout 4
Core			
1. Valslide mountain climber	2 × AMRAP		
Strength			
2a. Single-leg Romanian deadlift	2–3 × 12*		
2b. Push-up variation†	2–3 × 12		
3a. Front squat	2–3 × 12		
3b. Cable bent-over row (dual handles)	2–3 × 12		
Intervals			
	AMRAP × 85% MHR/65% MHR in 10 minutes‡		

AMRAP = as many reps as possible; *MHR* = maximum heart rate.

Suggested rest time between sets: up to 60 seconds.

* Each side.

† Use a different variation for each rep range.

‡ For explanation, see p. 66.

STAGE 5

Workout A: 2 and 5

Exercise	Sets × Reps	Workout 2	Workout 5 ⇨
Core			
1. Valslide mountain climber	2 × AMRAP		
Strength			
2a. Single-leg Romanian deadlift	3–4 × 8*		
2b. Push-up variation†	3–4 × 8		
3a. Front squat	3–4 × 8		
3b. Cable bent-over row (dual handles)	3–4 × 8		
Intervals			
	AMRAP × 85% MHR/65% MHR in 10 minutes‡		

AMRAP = as many reps as possible; *MHR* = maximum heart rate; ⇨ = rep out on final set of each strength exercise in Workout 5.

Suggested rest time between sets: 60–90 seconds.

* Each side.

† Use a different variation for each rep range.

‡ For explanation, see p. 66.

STAGE 5

Workout A: Workouts 3 and 6

Exercise	Sets × Reps	Workout 3	Workout 6
Core			
1. Valslide mountain climber	2 × AMRAP		
Strength			
2a. Single-leg Romanian deadlift	2–3 × 10*		
2b. Push-up variation†	2–3 × 10		
3a. Front squat	2–3 × 10		
3b. Cable bent-over row (dual handles)	2–3 × 10		
Intervals			
	AMRAP × 85% MHR/65% MHR in 10 minutes‡		

AMRAP = as many reps as possible; *MHR* = maximum heart rate.

Suggested rest time between sets: 60 seconds.

* Each side.

† Use a different variation for each rep range.

‡ For explanation, see p. 66.

STAGE 5

Workout B: Workouts 1 and 4

Exercise	Sets × Reps	Workout 1	Workout 4
Core			
1. Suspended fallout or rollout variation	2 × 12–15		
Strength			
2a. Reverse lunge	2–3 × 10*		
2b. Inverted row†	2–3 × 10		
3a. Kettlebell swing	2–3 × 10		
3b. Dumbbell single-arm push press	2–3 × 10*		
Intervals			
	AMRAP × 85% MHR/65% MHR in 10 minutes‡		

AMRAP = as many reps as possible; *MHR* = maximum heart rate.

Suggested rest time between sets: 60 seconds.

* Each side.

† Use a different grip and/or bar height for each rep range.

‡ For explanation, see p. 66.

STAGE 5

Workout B: 2 and 5

Exercise	Sets × Reps	Workout 2	Workout 5
Core			
1. Suspended fallout or rollout variation	2 × 12–15		
Strength			
2a. Reverse lunge	2–3 × 12*		
2b. Inverted row†	2–3 × 12		
3a. Kettlebell swing	2–3 × 12		
3b. Dumbbell single-arm push press	2–3 × 12*		
Intervals			
	AMRAP × 85% MHR/65% MHR in 10 minutes‡		

AMRAP = as many reps as possible; *MHR* = maximum heart rate.

Suggested rest time between sets: up to 60 seconds.

* Each side.

† Use a different grip and/or bar height for each rep range

‡ For explanation, see p. 66.

STAGE 5			
Workout B: 3 and 6			
Exercise	**Sets × Reps**	**Workout 3**	**Workout 6** ⇨
Core			
1. Suspended fallout or rollout variation	2 × 12–15		
Strength			
2a. Reverse lunge	3–4 × 8*		
2b. Inverted row‡	3–4 × 8		
3a. Kettlebell swing	3–4 × 8		
3b. Dumbbell single-arm push press	3–4 × 8*		
Intervals			
	AMRAP × 85% MHR/65% MHR in 10 minutes‡		

AMRAP = as many reps as possible; *MHR* = maximum heart rate; ⇨ = rep out on final set of each strength exercise in Workout 6.

Suggested rest time between sets: 60–90 seconds.

* Each side.

† Use a different grip and/or bar height for each rep range.

‡ For explanation, see p. 66.

STAGE 6

Here's what a month of training will look like:

	Monday	Tuesday	Wednesday	Thursday	Friday	Saturday	Sunday
Week 1	A: Workout 1 (3 × 8)	off	B: Workout 1 (4 × 4)	off	A: Workout 2 (3 × 6)	off	off
Week 2	B: Workout 2 (3 × 8)	off	A: Workout 3 (4 × 4)	off	B: Workout 3 (3 × 6)	off	off
Week 3	A: Workout 4 (3 × 8)	off	B: Workout 4 (4 × 4)	off	A: Workout 5 ⇨ (3 × 6)	off	off
Week 4	B: Workout 5 (3 × 8)	off	A: Workout 6 (4 × 4)	off	B: Workout 6 ⇨ (3 × 6)	off	off

THE KEY TO STAGE 6

The charts in Stage 6 show a fixed number of sets for each exercise, rather than "2–3" or "3–4." But the key to the program isn't the sets. It's the reps. When a workout calls for 3 × 8, think of that equation literally, as 24 reps. But these are 24 very specific reps. Same with the 18 reps when you do 3 × 6 and the 16 from 4 × 4.

When You Do 24 Reps (3 × 8):

You want to use a weight you're pretty sure you can lift 10 times in an all-out set. That weight will probably be 70 to 75 percent of your one-repetition max on that exercise.

When You Do 18 Reps (3 × 6):

Use a weight you think you can lift 8 times, which would be 75 to 80 percent of your one-rep max.

When You Do 16 Reps (4 × 4):

This weight should be about 85 percent of your max, which you could probably lift 6 times.

You want every rep to be a good one, with consistent form and lifting speed. To pull that off, expect to take more time between sets. That's the only way to reach the desired quantity with the mandatory quality.

STAGE 6

Workout A: 1 and 4

Exercise	Sets × Reps	Workout 1	Workout 4
Core			
1. Valslide Spider-Man push-away	6–8*		
2. Split-stance cable chop	2 × 12*		
Strength			
3a. Deadlift	3 × 8		
3b. Incline dumbbell or barbell bench press	3 × 8		
4a. Suspended lunge	3 × 8*		
4b. Dumbbell single-arm dead-stop row	3 × 8*		
Intervals			
	AMRAP × 85% MHR/65% MHR in 10 minutes†		

AMRAP = as many reps as possible; *MHR* = maximum heart rate.

Suggested rest time between sets: up to 60 seconds.

* Each side.

† For explanation, see p. 66.

STAGE 6

Workout A: 2 and 5

Exercise	Sets × Reps	Workout 2	Workout 5 ⇨
Core			
1. Valslide Spider-Man push-away	6–8*		
2. Split-stance cable chop	2 × 12*		
Strength			
3a. Deadlift	4 × 4		
3b. Incline dumbbell or barbell bench press	4 × 4		
4a. Suspended lunge	4 × 4*		
4b. Dumbbell single-arm dead-stop row	4 × 4*		
Intervals			
	AMRAP × 85% MHR/65% MHR in 10 minutes†		

AMRAP = as many reps as possible; *MHR* = maximum heart rate; ⇨ = rep out on final set of each strength exercise in Workout 5.

Suggested rest time between sets: 60–90 seconds.

* Each side.

† For explanation, see p. 66.

STAGE 6

Workout A: 3 and 6

Exercise	Sets × Reps	Workout 3	Workout 6
Core			
1. Valslide Spider-Man push-away	6–8*		
2. Split-stance cable chop	2 × 12*		
Strength			
3a. Deadlift	3 × 6		
3b. Incline dumbbell or barbell bench press	3 × 6		
4a. Suspended lunge	3 × 6*		
4b. Dumbbell single-arm dead-stop row	3 × 6*		
Intervals			
	AMRAP × 85% MHR/65% MHR in 10 minutes†		

AMRAP = as many reps as possible; *MHR* = maximum heart rate.

Suggested rest time between sets: 60 seconds.

* Each side.

† For explanation, see p. 66.

STAGE 6

Workout B: 1 and 4

Exercise	Sets × Reps	Workout 1	Workout 4
Core			
1. Suspended jackknife	2 × 10		
2. Split-stance cable lift	2 × 10*		
Strength			
3a. Back squat to box with pause	3 × 6		
3b. Chin-up or band-assisted chin-up	3 × 6		
4a. Rear-foot-elevated split squat	3 × 6*		
4b. Dumbbell neutral-grip bench press	3 × 6		
Intervals			
	AMRAP × 85% MHR/65% MHR in 10 minutes†		

AMRAP = as many reps as possible; *MHR* = maximum heart rate.

Suggested rest time between sets: 60 seconds.

* Each side.

† For explanation, see p. 66.

STAGE 6

Workout B: 2 and 5

Exercise	Sets/Reps	Workout 2	Workout 5
Core			
1. Suspended jackknife	2 × 10		
2. Split-stance cable lift	2 × 10*		
Strength			
3a. Back squat to box with pause	3 × 8		
3b. Chin-up or band-assisted chin-up	3 × 8		
4a. Rear-foot-elevated split squat	3 × 8*		
4b. Dumbbell neutral-grip bench press	3 × 8		
Intervals			
	AMRAP × 85% MHR/65% MHR in 10 minutes†		

AMRAP = as many reps as possible; *MHR* = maximum heart rate.

Suggested rest time between sets: 60 seconds.

* Each side.

† For explanation, see p. 66.

STAGE 6

Workout B: 3 and 6

Exercise	Sets × Reps	Workout 3	Workout 6 ⇨
Core			
1. Suspended jackknife	2 × 10		
2. Split-stance cable lift	2 × 10*		
Strength			
3a. Back squat to box with pause	4 × 4		
3b. Chin-up or band-assisted chin-up	4 × 4		
4a. Rear-foot-elevated split squat	4 × 4*		
4b. Dumbbell neutral-grip bench press	4 × 4		
Intervals			
	AMRAP × 85% MHR/65% MHR in 10 minutes†		

AMRAP = as many reps as possible; *MHR* = maximum heart rate; ⇨ = rep out on final set of each strength exercise in Workout 6.

Suggested rest time between sets: 60 seconds.

* Each side.

† For explanation, see p. 66.

Phase Three: Display

THE LONGER YOU TRAIN, AND THE more adaptations you make to training, the better you appreciate a fundamental truth: Your performance potential changes slightly from workout to workout. The more you focus on strength, with heavier weights and higher value assigned to each set, the more it comes into play. There are days when a near-maximum weight will go up easily, and days when it will barely move. It's hard not to feel like a failure when you struggle. But pushing yourself past your limits on those rough days is a good way to induce an injury.

Fortunately, there's a middle ground in between "I suck" and "I'm hurt." Some of the strongest people in the world have rethought the numbers-focused paradigm and shifted the emphasis to effort, an idea we've embraced in *Strong*. The goal of each workout is to reach a predetermined *rate of perceived exertion* (RPE), rather than a specific load. Here's how it looks as a scale from 1 to 10.

RPE	What it feels like
1	Nothing
2	Lifting your arms or legs, barely feeling the effects of gravity
3	A movement you do on purpose, like a mobility exercise in RAMP
4	Still easy, something you'd have to do at least 20 times to exhaust your muscles
5	Your first warm-up set; you could easily do twice as many reps
6	Your second warm-up set; it's starting to feel like work, but not close to a maximum effort
7	Your final warm-up or first work set
8	Most lifters, most of the time, end sets here, when they could do at least 2 more reps
9	A very difficult set; at most, you could do one more rep
10	An all-out set, the most reps you can do that day, with that weight

Pay the most attention to RPE 8, 9, and 10. Those are the levels of effort Alwyn prescribes in Phase Three, which, as promised, is very different from the previous phases.

WORKOUTS A, B, AND C

Instead of alternating Workout A and Workout B, you'll do three different workouts. Ideally, you'll do each of them once a week for four weeks. That's why, in the charts, you'll see columns for Week 1, Week 2, etc., instead of Workout 1 and Workout 2.

FEATURED STRENGTH EXERCISE

Phase One and Phase Two put equal emphasis on the four strength exercises in each workout, with the same sets and reps. In Phase Three your primary focus will be on one featured exercise:

Workout A: squat
Workout B: press
Workout C: deadlift

You decide which version you do within each movement pattern. The obvious choices are the three powerlifts: barbell back squat, barbell bench press, and either traditional or sumo-style deadlifts. Or you can go with exercises you'll never see in a competition, like goblet squats, dumbbell shoulder presses, and hex-bar deadlifts. As long as it allows you to do low-rep sets with maximal weights, it can work.

You also have the choice of using the same exercises in each stage or trying different ones. If your goal is to finish Phase Three with your all-time best lifts, you probably want to use the same ones in all three stages. But you don't have to do it that way. Personally, I know my best lifts are deep in the rearview mirror, and that I'm far less likely to exceed them than I am to injure myself trying. For me, it's more interesting and fun to see what I can do with several different variations.

THE OTHER STRENGTH EXERCISES

Following your sets with the featured exercise, you'll do four more exercises the traditional way, as alternating sets: 2a and 2b, followed by 3a and 3b. How you do them will change from stage to stage, which I'll explain when we get there. As always, you want to challenge yourself with these exercises, with the goal of improving your performance from week to week.

CORE EXERCISES

Core training in Phase Two was complex and exhausting. It was like having six or seven strength exercises per workout, instead of four. Now you're going to dial it back to one core exercise per workout. They're all tough exercises. But they're also kind of fun if you like a challenge. (And if you don't like a challenge, you won't have to worry because you aren't going to last long in Phase Three.)

INTERVALS

Alwyn doesn't prescribe intervals in Phase Three. There's enough fatigue built into the strength program; adding more with intervals might inhibit your recovery from workout to workout. If you feel you need some type of cardio training, Alwyn recommends doing intervals once a week on a nonlifting day, perhaps for 20 to 30 minutes at most.

STAGE 7

Workout A

Exercise	Sets × Reps	Week 1	Week 2	Week 3	Week 4
Core					
1. Suspended body saw	1–2 × 8–12				
Strength					
		RPE 8	RPE 9	RPE 10	*
2. Squat[†]	Work up to top set of 5 reps				
3a. Pull (horizontal)	2–3 × 10				
3b. Single-leg Romanian deadlift	2–3 × 10[‡]				
4a. Push-up or press	2–3 × 10				
4b. Supine hip extension + leg curl	2–3 × 10				

RPE = rate of perceived exertion.

Suggested rest time between sets: 2–3 minutes for squats, 60 seconds for following exercises.

* Following a warm-up set, do 2 sets of 5 with 70–75 percent of the weight you used in Week 3. Aim for an RPE of 7.

[†] Alwyn recommends the barbell front squat.

[‡] Each side.

STAGE 7

Workout B

Exercise	Sets × Reps	Week 1	Week 2	Week 3	Week 4
Core					
1. Suspended pike	1–2 × 8–12				
Strength					
		RPE 8	RPE 9	RPE 10	*
2. Press[†]	Work up to top set of 5 reps				
3a. Lunge	2–3 × 10[‡]				
3b. Pull (vertical)	2–3 × 10				
4a. Squat	2–3 × 10				
4b. Pull (horizontal)	2–3 × 10				

RPE = rate of perceived exertion.

Suggested rest time between sets: 2–3 minutes for presses, 60 seconds for following exercises.

* Following a warm-up set, do 2 sets of 5 with 70–75 percent of the weight you used in Week 3. Aim for an RPE of 7.

[†] Alwyn recommends the barbell shoulder press

[‡] Each side.

STAGE 7					
Workout C					
Exercise	Sets × Reps	Week 1	Week 2	Week 3	Week 4
Core					
1. Standing antirotation press + overhead raise	1–2 × 8–12				
Strength					
		RPE 8	RPE 9	RPE 10	*
2. Deadlift	Work up to top set of 5 reps				
3a. Push-up or press	2–3 × 10				
3b. Lunge	2–3 × 10†				
4a. Pull (vertical)	2–3 × 10				
4b. Step-up	2–3 × 10				

RPE = rate of perceived exertion.

Suggested rest time between sets: 2–3 minutes for deadlifts, 60 seconds for following exercises.

* Following a warm-up set, do 2 sets of 5 with 70–75 percent of the weight you used in Week 3. Aim for an RPE of 7.

† Each side.

HOW TO DO THE FEATURED EXERCISE

We'll start with the squat in Workout A. Alwyn recommends the barbell front squat for Stage 7, but as mentioned earlier, it's really up to you. Once you decide on a variation, do this:

Week 1

1. Select a weight you think you can lift at least 10 times. Do 5 reps.
2. Add 5 pounds. Do 5 reps.
3. Add another 5 pounds. Do 5 reps.
4. Continue until you reach RPE 8 on a set of 5 reps. You should finish this set feeling as if you could have done two more.

Four more guidelines:

• Aim for a total of 5 sets, although it's not a problem if you hit your RPE target on the fourth set, or if you need more than 5.

- Stronger and more experienced lifters may need to add more than 5 pounds per set.
- Record each set. If you went over the recommended 5 sets, you probably need to start with a heavier weight on your first set, and/or make bigger jumps from set to set. If you reached RPE 8 before your fifth set, you probably need to do the opposite: Start lighter and/or increase the weight in smaller increments.
- Rest as long as you need between sets. If you're an impatient type (like me), make yourself wait a little longer than you normally would.

Week 2

Do the exact same thing, but now you want to reach RPE 9 on that final set of 5 reps. It should feel as if you could *maybe* get one more rep. Once again, aim for 5 total sets.

Week 3

By now you should have a pretty good idea of how to reach RPE 10 by your final set. If you get to your fifth set with a little left in the tank, no problem. Add a little weight to the bar, take a long rest (at least 3 minutes), and then go for that perfect 10. It's okay if you get only 4 reps instead of 5.

Week 4

This is your recovery week. Pull out your calculator, and multiply the weight you used in your final set in Week 3 by 0.75. That's the weight you'll use for 2 easy sets of 5 reps, following a warm-up set.

HOW TO DO THE NEXT FOUR EXERCISES

You also have some leeway in selecting the rest of your exercises. In most slots, Alwyn specifies the movement pattern—lunge, step-up, push-up or press, vertical or horizontal pull—and you decide which variation makes the most sense for you. Some tips and guidelines:

Pulling Exercises

When you look at one of Alwyn's programs, you expect to see an equal emphasis on upper-body pushing and pulling exercises. But with a quick glance at Stage 7, you'll see that there's no equivalent to the press in Workout B. Instead, two of the next four exercises are pulls—one horizontal (a row), one vertical (a chin-up or lat pulldown). You'll also see a horizontal row in Workout A and a vertical row in Workout C.

Although it's your choice, here are our recommendations:

Workout A (horizontal): cable row, or the equivalent with a resistance band. Squats, the featured exercise, force your lower-back muscles to work hard to keep your lower back and pelvis in a safe, neutral position. Doing rows with a barbell or dumbbell might be too much stress on those same muscles for one workout.

Workout B (vertical): chin-up or inverted row. Whichever of these you can manage for 10 reps will be a perfect complement for the press, the featured exercise.

Workout B (horizontal): dumbbell row. Pick the variation you think is most productive for you.

Workout C (vertical): lat pulldown. What I just said about the squat fatiguing your lower-back muscles goes double for the deadlift. But it's not just the obvious core muscles that get worked. Your lats are key muscles in the deadlift; they not only help stabilize your lower back but help control the barbell as you pull it up from the floor. The heavier the bar, the more work they do. The pulldown is a nice complement, in that it works the lats through a full range of motion without putting the lower back at risk.

Press

You can use either type as the featured exercise in Workout B. Alwyn prefers the shoulder press, but many of you will choose the bench press because it's one of the three powerlifts. (The shoulder press used to be part of Olympic weightlifting. By the time it was dropped, after the 1972 games, it didn't look anything like the exercise we do today.) For either, you probably want to use a barbell, rather than dumbbells. Dumbbells force you to increase the weight by 10 pounds at a time (5 pounds per dumbbell), but you can advance 5 pounds at a time with a barbell, if you have 2.5-pound plates. If your gym has 1.25-pound plates ("Cheerios," in gym parlance), you can add just 2.5 pounds per set.

In workouts A and C, you'll see "push-up or press" following the featured exercise. Select a variation that's different from the press in Workout B. If you use the shoulder press as your featured exercise, you probably want to do push-up and bench press variations in A and C. If you use the bench press in B, you can do the shoulder press and incline bench press in the other two workouts.

STAGE 8

The structure of the program in Stage 8 is the same as Stage 7. You still have three workouts—A, B, and C—and each workout progresses the same way, with a core exercise followed by the five strength exercises. But there are big changes to the way you do the strength program.

HOW TO DO THE FEATURED EXERCISE

In Week 3 of Stage 7, you reached a 5-rep max in each of the featured exercises. For Stage 8, you need to begin with your 10-rep max, which should be about 85 percent of your 5-rep max. So if you used 100 pounds for 5 reps, you can assume your 10-rep max is 85 pounds. Here's what you'll do with it.

Week 1

Start with a warm-up set. Do 5 reps with a weight that's probably two-thirds to three-quarters of your 10-rep max. If your 10-rep max is 85 pounds, you want to do your warm-up set with 55 to 65 pounds. (There's no magic formula for a warm-up set. All you're doing is practicing the movement and preparing your body without exhausting your muscles.)

Now do sets of 5, 4, and 3 reps with your 10-rep max, resting as much as you need in between. (Alwyn recommends 90 seconds.) Then move on to the next four exercises. Before you ask the obvious question—"Wait, that's it?"—keep in mind that you're doing 12 reps with your 10-rep max. That's the key.

Week 2

Do a warm-up, as described. Add 5 to 10 pounds to the weights you used in Week 1 (probably 10 pounds for squats and deadlifts and 5 pounds for presses), and do the same thing: sets of 5, 4, and 3 reps.

This time, you're doing 12 reps with a weight that, in all likelihood, is more than 90 percent of the 5-rep max you established in Stage 7.

Week 3

Same steps: Do 1 or 2 warm-up sets. Add 5 to 10 pounds to your Week 2 weights. Do sets of 5, 4, and 3+ reps. If you can't get more than 3, that's great—it means you're working with the heaviest weights possible. But if you still have something in the tank after your third one, keep going until you squeeze out every possible repetition.

Your goal is to do at least 12 reps with what used to be your 5-rep max . . . which is no longer your *true* 5-rep max because you're stronger now.

Week 4

Recovery week: Do 2 to 3 easy sets of 5 reps, aiming for an RPE around 7.

HOW TO DO THE NEXT FOUR EXERCISES

Instead of giving you three different combinations of exercises, one each for Workouts A, B, and C, Alwyn gives you two: In the first you'll do 2 to 3 sets of 8 reps. In the second you'll do 2 to 3 sets of 12. You'll alternate between them. For someone who trains on Monday, Wednesday, and Friday, a month of workouts will look like this:

	Monday	**Wednesday**	**Friday**
Week 1	Workout A Featured: squat Others: 2–3 × 8	Workout B Featured: press Others: 2–3 × 12	Workout C Featured: deadlift Others: 2–3 × 8
Week 2	Workout A Featured: squat Others: 2–3 × 12	Workout B Featured: press Others: 2–3 × 8	Workout C Featured: deadlift Others: 2–3 × 12
Week 3	Workout A Featured: squat Others: 2–3 × 8	Workout B Featured: press Others: 2–3 × 12	Workout C Featured: deadlift Others: 2–3 × 8
Week 4	Workout A Featured: squat Others: 2–3 × 12	Workout B Featured: press Others: 2–3 × 8	Workout C Featured: deadlift Others: 2–3 × 12

Again, you want to work hard on these exercises, but you don't want to push yourself to complete muscular exhaustion on any sets. Don't worry if it happens by accident; you never know how your effort on the featured exercise will affect the rest of the workout. Just don't make it your goal to train to failure on these exercises.

STAGE 8

Workout A

Exercise	Sets × Reps	Week 1	Week 2	Week 3	Week 4
Core					
1. Ab-wheel rollout	1–2 × 8–10				
Strength					
		10 RM	+5–10 lb.	+5–10 lb.#	*
2. Squat	3 × 5, 4, 3				
Alternate the following two combinations of exercises, as shown in the chart on p. 97.					
First Combination					
3a. Pull (horizontal)	2–3 × 8				
3b. Lunge	2–3 × 8†				
4a. Push-up or press	2–3 × 8				
4b. Single-leg hip thrust	2–3 × 8†				
Second Combination					
3a. Push-up or press‡	2–3 × 12				
3b. Single-leg Romanian deadlift	2–3 × 12†				
4a. Pull (vertical)	2–3 × 12				
4b. Lunge‡	2–3 × 12†				

10 RM = your 10-rep max, which should be about 85 percent of the 5-rep max you established in Stage 7.

Suggested rest time between sets: 90 seconds for squats, 60 seconds for all other exercises.

* After a warm-up set, do 2–3 easy sets of 5. Aim for an RPE of 7.

† Each side.

‡ Choose a different variation from the one you used for 8 reps per set.

Do 3+ reps on final set.

STAGE 8

Workout B

Exercise	Sets × Reps	Week 1	Week 2	Week 3	Week 4
Core					
1. Hanging knee raise	1–2 × 8–10				
Strength					
		10 RM	+5–10 lb.	+5–10 lb.#	*
2. Press	3 × 5, 4, 3				
Alternate the following two combinations of exercises, as shown in the chart on p. 97.					
First Combination					
3a. Pull (horizontal)	2–3 × 8				
3b. Lunge	2–3 × 8†				
4a. Push-up or press‡	2–3 × 8				
4b. Single-leg hip thrust	2–3 × 8†				
Second Combination					
3a. Push-up or press‡	2–3 × 12				
3b. Single-leg Romanian deadlift	2–3 × 12†				
4a. Pull (vertical)	2–3 × 12				
4b. Lunge§	2–3 × 12†				

10 RM = your 10-rep max, which should be about 85 percent of the 5-rep max you established in Stage 7.

Suggested rest time between sets: 90 seconds for presses, 60 seconds for following exercises.

* After a warm-up set, do 2–3 easy sets of 5. Aim for an RPE of 7.

† Each side.

‡ In both exercise combinations (8 and 12 reps per set) choose a different variation from your featured exercise. So if you do the barbell shoulder press, you might choose the dumbbell bench press for sets of 8 reps and a push-up or cable chest press for sets of 12.

§ Choose a different variation from the one you used for 8 reps per set.

Do 3+ reps on final set.

STAGE 8

Workout C

Exercise	Sets × Reps	Week 1	Week 2	Week 3	Week 4
Core					
1. Cable horizontal chop	1–2 × 8–10				
Strength					
		10 RM	+5–10 lb.	+5–10 lb.#	*
2. Deadlift	3 × 5, 4, 3				
Alternate the following two combinations of exercises, as shown in the chart on p. 97.					
First Combination					
3a. Pull (horizontal)	2–3 × 8				
3b. Lunge	2–3 × 8†				
4a. Push-up or press	2–3 × 8				
4b. Single-leg hip thrust	2–3 × 8†				
Second Combination					
3a. Push-up or press‡	2–3 × 12				
3b. Single-leg Romanian deadlift	2–3 × 12†				
4a. Pull (vertical)	2–3 × 12				
4b. Lunge‡	2–3 × 12†				

10 RM = your 10-rep max, which should be about 85 percent of the 5-rep max you established in Stage 7.

Suggested rest time between sets: 90 seconds for squats, 60 seconds for following exercises.

* After a warm-up set, do 2–3 easy sets of 5. Aim for an RPE of 7.

† Each side.

‡ Choose a different variation from the one you used for 8 reps per set.

Do 3+ reps on final set.

STAGE 9

We now come to the final stage in *Strong*, and a training technique that may very well be the toughest in any of the six books featuring Alwyn's programs. These workouts employ *drop sets*, a trick used for many years, in many ways, by body builders. The process is simple enough: For any exercise, you would do a set to failure, drop the weight, do another set to failure, and repeat until the targeted muscles have reached the deepest possible level of exhaustion.

These drop sets are similar in execution, but different in purpose. You do them with only the three featured exercises—squat, press, deadlift—which means your focus is on the movement pattern, rather than individual muscles. You also use progressively heavier weights each week, with fewer repetitions. This imposes a tremendous amount of systemic stress, designed to trigger a potentially dramatic metabolic response.

HOW TO DO THE FEATURED EXERCISE

How you do the drop sets will differ slightly each week:

Week 1

1. Work up to a 7-rep max (as described on p. 96)
2. Strip about 10 percent of the weight from the bar.
3. Do as many reps as possible.
4. Strip another 10 percent from the bar.
5. Do as many reps as possible.

A few tips:

- For your 7-rep max, you want to hit an RPE between 9 and 10. At most, you could maybe get one more rep. For the 2 drop sets, your goal is RPE 10. Don't leave anything in the tank.
- Rest as much as you need while working up to your 7-rep max. Then take 30 seconds in between drop sets, which should be about the time it takes you to reduce the weight by 10 percent.
- Don't worry about getting exactly 10 percent on each drop. Math is hard to do without oxygen in your brain. Just get close and go. The following is a practical example.
  - Let's say your 7-rep max for the deadlift is 135 pounds. That's an Olympic barbell (usually 45 pounds) and a 45-pound plate on each side. Ten percent is 13.5 pounds, which means you have 30 seconds to strip the bar down to 121.5 pounds. In most circumstances, the best you can do is 120 pounds: the bar (45 pounds), two 25-pound plates (one on each side), two 10-pound plates, and two 2.5-pound plates. If you also happen to have a pair of 1.25-pound plates, you can hit 121.5 on the nose. But unless you have two spotters to help you and have gathered up all the aforementioned plates before starting, it's going to take longer than 30 seconds to put it together.

    Then you have to take another 10 percent off for the second and final drop set, which would be 12 pounds (or 12.15, if you managed to use exactly 121.5 for the first drop set). It hurts my brain to think of how to configure 108 pounds on an Olympic bar. So in that circumstance I'd use 105: the bar, two 25-pounders, and two 5-pounders. I could do that in 30 seconds without straining any cognitive neurons.

Week 2

Work up to a 5-rep max, and then repeat the process: strip 10 percent of the weight, do as many reps as possible, strip another 10 percent, and rep out again.

Week 3

Do the same thing, only this time with a 3-rep max.

Week 4

Do 2 to 3 sets of 5 reps with your 7-rep max from Week 1.

HOW TO DO THE NEXT FOUR EXERCISES

Instead of alternating rep ranges from one workout to the next, as you did in Stage 8, you'll alternate from week to week. It looks like this:

Weeks 1 and 3

2 to 3 sets of 6 reps

Weeks 2 and 4

2 to 3 sets of 10 reps

EXERCISE SELECTION

Although you'll see some specific exercises suggested, you shouldn't feel bound to them. The key is to stay true to the movement categories, to get as much variety as you need, and to avoid excessive stress on your most vulnerable areas—shoulders, knees, and lower back.

STAGE 9

Workout A, Week 1

Exercise	Sets × Reps			
Core				
1. Dumbbell plank row	1–2 × 8–10*			
Strength				
		7 RM	**Drop Set 1**	**Drop Set 2**
2. Squat				
3a. Pull (horizontal)	2–3 × 6*			
3b. Split stance†	2–3 × 6*			
4a. Push-up or press	2–3 × 6			
4b. Single leg†	2–3 × 6*			

7 RM = your 7-rep max, which should be about 95 percent of the 5-rep max you established in Stage 8.

* Each side.

† Your choice of any exercise in this category.

STAGE 9

Workout A, Week 2

Exercise	Sets × Reps			
Core				
1. Dumbbell plank row	1–2 × 8–10*			
Strength				
		5 RM	**Drop Set 1**	**Drop Set 2**
2. Squat				
3a. Push-up or press	2–3 × 10*			
3b. Single leg†	2–3 × 10*			
4a. Pull (horizontal)	2–3 × 10			
4b. Split stance†	2–3 × 10*			

5 RM = your 5-rep max, which should be about 5 percent more than the 7-rep max you achieved in Week 1.

* Each side.

† Your choice of any exercise in this category.

STAGE 9

Workout A, Week 3

Exercise	Sets × Reps			
Core				
1. Dumbbell plank row	1–2 × 8–10*			
Strength				
		3 RM	**Drop Set 1**	**Drop Set 2**
2. Squat				
3a. Pull (horizontal)	2–3 × 6*			
3b. Split stance†	2–3 × 6*			
4a. Push-up or press	2–3 × 6			
4b. Single leg†	2–3 × 6*			

3 RM = your 3-rep max, which should be 5 to 7 percent more than the 5-rep max you achieved in Week 2.

* Each side.

† Your choice of any exercise in this category.

STAGE 9

Workout A, Week 4

Exercise	Sets × Reps			
Core				
1. Dumbbell plank row	1–2 × 8–10*			
Strength				
2. Squat	2–3 × 5†			
3a. Push-up or press	2–3 × 10*			
3b. Single leg‡	2–3 × 10*			
4a. Pull (horizontal)	2–3 × 10			
4b. Split stance‡	2–3 × 10*			

* Each side.

† For all sets, use the 7 RM weight from Week 1.

‡ Your choice of any exercise in this category.

STAGE 9

Workout B, Week 1

Exercise	Sets × Reps	7 RM	Drop Set 1	Drop Set 2
Core				
1. Windmill	1–2 × 5–8*			
Strength				
2. Press				
3a. Pull (vertical)	2–3 × 6			
3b. Split stance†	2–3 × 6*			
4a. Push-up or press	2–3 × 6			
4b. Single leg†	2–3 × 6*			

7 RM = your 7-rep max, which should be about 95 percent of the 5-rep max you established in Stage 8.

* Each side.

† Your choice of any exercise in this category.

STAGE 9

Workout B, Week 2

Exercise	Sets × Reps	5 RM	Drop Set 1	Drop Set 2
Core				
1. Windmill	1–2 × 5–8*			
Strength				
2. Press				
3a. Push-up or press	2–3 × 10			
3b. Single leg†	2–3 × 10*			
4a. Pull (vertical)	2–3 × 10			
4b. Split stance†	2–3 × 10*			

5 RM = your 5-rep max, which should be about 5 percent more than the 7-rep max you achieved in Week 1.

* Each side.

† Your choice of any exercise in this category.

STAGE 9

Workout B, Week 3

Exercise	Sets × Reps			
Core				
1. Windmill	1–2 × 5–8*			
Strength				
		3 RM	Drop Set 1	Drop Set 2
2. Press				
3a. Pull (vertical)	2–3 × 6			
3b. Split stance†	2–3 × 6*			
4a. Push-up or press	2–3 × 6			
4b. Single leg†	2–3 × 6*			

3 RM = your 3-rep max, which should be 5 to 7 percent more than the 5-rep max you achieved in Week 2.

* Each side.

† Your choice of any exercise in this category.

STAGE 9

Workout B, Week 4

Exercise	Sets × Reps			
Core				
1. Windmill	1–2 × 5–8*			
Strength				
2. Press	2–3 × 5†			
3a. Push-up or press	2–3 × 10			
3b. Single leg‡	2–3 × 10*			
4a. Pull (vertical)	2–3 × 10			
4b. Split stance‡	2–3 × 10*			

* Each side.

† For all sets, use the 7 RM weight from Week 1.

‡ Your choice of any exercise in this category.

STAGE 9

Workout C, Week 1

Exercise	Sets × Reps			
Core				
1. Cable high to low chop	1–2 × 10*			
Strength				
		7 RM	**Drop Set 1**	**Drop Set 2**
2. Deadlift				
3a. Inverted row	2–3 × 6			
3b. Split stance†	2–3 × 6*			
4a. Push-up or press	2–3 × 6			
4b. Single leg†	2–3 × 6*			

7 RM = your 7-rep max, which should be about 95 percent of the 5-rep max you established in Stage 8.

* Each side.

† Your choice of any exercise in this category.

STAGE 9

Workout C, Week 2

Exercise	Sets × Reps			
Core				
1. Cable high to low chop	1–2 x 10*			
Strength				
		5 RM	**Drop Set 1**	**Drop Set 2**
2. Deadlift				
3a. Push-up or press	2–3 × 10			
3b. Single leg†	2–3 × 10*			
4a. Inverted row	2–3 × 10			
4b. Split stance†	2–3 × 10*			

5 RM = your 5-rep max, which should be about 5 percent more than the 7-rep max you achieved in Week 1.

* Each side.

† Your choice of any exercise in this category.

STAGE 9

Workout C, Week 3

Exercise	Sets × Reps			
Core				
1. Cable high to low chop	1–2 × 10*			
Strength				
		3 RM	**Drop Set 1**	**Drop Set 2**
2. Deadlift				
3a. Inverted row	2–3 × 6			
3b. Split stance†	2–3 × 6*			
4a. Push-up or press	2–3 × 6			
4b. Single leg†	2–3 × 6*			

3 RM = your 3-rep max, which should be 5 to 7 percent more than the 5-rep max you achieved in Week 2.

* Each side.

† Your choice of any exercise in this category.

STAGE 9

Workout C, Week 4

Exercise	Sets × Reps			
Core				
1. Cable high to low chop	1–2 x 10*			
Strength				
2. Deadlift	2–3 × 5†			
3a. Push-up or press	2–3 × 10			
3b. Single leg‡	2–3 × 10*			
4a. Inverted row	2–3 × 10			
4b. Split stance‡	2–3 × 10*			

* Each side.

† For all sets, use the 7 RM weight from Week 1.

‡ Your choice of any exercise in this category.

PART 3

The Exercises

Moves
That Matter

MOST WORKOUTS ARE BASED ON EXERCISES. The goal of each exercise, most of the time, is to work specific muscles. It's the most instinctive way to train. You want bigger biceps, so you do exercises that clearly, unambiguously squeeze your biceps. Or you want shapelier thighs, so you do lunges, which clearly, unambiguously stretch and flex those muscles.

Alwyn has a different approach, as most of you understand by now. He starts with basic human movement patterns: running, jumping, climbing, throwing, lifting, carrying. Then he finds the right exercises for those patterns, with an understanding of what needs to move, how it needs to move, and just as important, what needs to *not* move.

If it's a good workout, one that helps you reach your goals, the philosophy behind it doesn't matter all that much. Human movements evolved along with human muscles. Muscles facilitate movements, and movements employ muscles. The two are inseparable. It doesn't matter if you do squats and deadlifts to build total-body strength and power, or to develop specific muscles in your back, hips, and thighs. As long as you do squats and deadlifts in a way that allows you to get stronger and more skilled over time, the results should be exactly the same.

That said, if you struggle with a particular exercise, it helps to understand that *the exercise itself* is never the goal. My friend Nick Tumminello has a great piece of advice: Don't fit your body to the exercise; fit the exercise to your body. The barbell back squat is a perfect example. Even when I could do it with moderately heavy weights, it took me a full week to recover. My knees felt like I'd hit them with hammers for the first few days. I tried to return to them a couple of times, but the results were even worse; now my back, hips, *and* knees felt mauled.

Fortunately, there are lots of ways to work the same movement pattern. At first it surprised me that I could do a front squat or goblet squat and feel as if I'd gotten a better workout with a completely pain-free range of motion. Now I don't really think about it. I use the exercises that allow me to work hardest with the least discomfort, during or after training, and enjoy the most benefits.

The emphasis on movement patterns applies to every part of the program. You'll find them all pictured and described in this order:

- RAMP (Chapter 11)
- Core training (Chapter 12)
- Squats, deadlifts, split-stance, and single-leg exercises (Chapter 13)
- Upper-body pushing and pulling exercises (Chapter 14)
- Interval training options (Chapter 15)

  Chapter 15 also includes some guidelines and suggestions for balancing sports and other types of training with the *Strong* program.

RAMP

The classic idea of a warm-up, which is still sometimes used in research, is a fixed amount of time on a treadmill or stationary bike. I'm sure it's a fine way to raise your core temperature, and it probably increases adrenaline as well. But in the same 10 minutes you might spend on a cardio machine, you can do a lot more than that.

That's the idea behind Alwyn's RAMP.

RAMP, as you may recall from Chapter 6, stands for range of motion, activation of muscles, and movement preparation. You can work on all that while also raising your core temperature slightly and generating a bit of adrenaline, which literally pumps you up for your workout by dilating blood vessels so more nutrients can reach your working muscles. A great warm-up routine should do all those things without exhausting the energy you'll need for the subsequent workout.

Here's a quick look at a sample RAMP session, in chart form.

Category	Examples	Reps/time/distance
Self-myofascial release, "hot spot" focus	• Foam rolling • Trigger-point pressure with ball • Targeted stretches	As needed on 5 areas (can also do this at end of workout)
Breathing reset	• Supine • Supine 90/90 with feet on wall • Prone "crocodile breathing" • Child's pose	5 deep breaths
Hip mobility	• Hip-flexor stretch with glute activation • Brettzel	30 seconds each side
Glute activation	• Hip raise • Single-leg hip raise • Marching hip raise	10–15 (with both legs), or 8–10 each side
Hip and upper-back mobility	• Child's pose with rotation • Spider-Man climb with reach	5–8 each side
Scapular stability	• Wall slide	8–10
Ankle mobility	• Single-leg calf stretch from push-up position	3–5 each side
Hip stability	• Clamshell • Walk with mini band	8–10 each side
Squat	• Squat to stand • Nose-to-wall squat	8–10
Single-leg balance, hip separation	• Walking knee hug, lunge, reach	6–8 each side
Hip separation, lateral movement	• Walking side lunge	6–8 each side
Forward or lateral movement, quick pace	• Jog • Side shuffle • Carioca • Jumping jack • Mountain climber	2 runs of 10–20 yards

There are two ways to use the information that follows.

- Ignore the explanations, and just do the first exercise in each category. You won't miss out on any benefits.
- Read the explanations so you understand the goal of each RAMP part. That way you can swap in exercises that accomplish the same things and personalize this part of the workout. Our selection only hints at the universe of options you have; Alwyn and his trainers know and incorporate more than we could ever list.

You can also abbreviate the warm-up for those times when you're rushed or during the summer when your core temperature rises faster and you walk into the weight room feeling limber and ready to work. At the opposite extreme, if you're a rapidly calcifying fossil like me, you can expand RAMP to address problem areas.

1. SELF-MYOFASCIAL RELEASE, "HOT SPOT" FOCUS

Most of you know what a foam roller is: a cylinder that's usually 6 inches wide and 18 to 36 inches long. You use it to apply pressure to potentially tight or stiff muscles, and to the fascia encasing them. In theory, this targeted compression helps break up the microscopic adhesions that bind tissues together and prevent them from playing nicely with each other. Is that actually how it works? Believe it or not, nobody knows. (Or at least, nobody can say for sure as I write this.)

Same with stretching. For a long time nobody knew for certain what stretching does to increase your range of motion. Researchers now believe it works by decreasing the sensation that the muscle is being stretched. When your connective tissues sense risk, they send an SOS to your brain. If you react in time, you'll prevent the type of injury caused by overstretching. By contrast, if you actually pull a muscle, the first thing you notice is that it gets tight. The range of motion shrinks to prevent further injury.

With both stretching and foam rolling, the goal is to convince your body to allow a greater, or less impeded, range of motion. They both seem to do that, and in one recent study, the two worked synergistically to increase hip flexibility to a greater extent than either alone.

Alwyn recommends using a foam roller to address five groups of muscles, with special focus on any "hot spots"—places in a muscle belly that, when compressed, produce acute but unexplainable pain. (*Explainable* pain includes an area that's bruised, scraped, or otherwise injured; you don't want to inflict foam rolling on a contusion.)

In the following pages we show the most common areas to roll out: glutes, hamstrings, iliotibial (IT) band, quads, and calves. You can also work on the lower back and lats. If you find a hot spot, a lacrosse ball may give you better results than a foam roller because all the compression can be concentrated on a small area.

In recent years I've added hamstring stretches to my warm-up, right after foam rolling and before the other exercises. They seem to help.

✳ Foam Rolling

- Work each area for 10 to 20 seconds, spending more time on areas that feel tighter than usual.
- Always roll in the direction of the muscle fibers, whether it's up and down or side to side.
- You have to relax the muscle completely to get the full effect, which can be tricky when you're tensing other muscles for balance or leverage. If you've never done it before, it might take a few tries before you get the hang of it.

✳ Trigger-Point Pressure with Ball

- When you find a trigger point—a spot within a muscle that's tender for no known reason—target it directly with something round and solid, like a lacrosse ball. Apply as much pressure as you can stand for 20 to 30 seconds.
- There's no need to go on search-and-destroy missions to find trigger points that pose no problems. This is one of those masochistic things some trainers do. (Mostly, I suspect, because they have a lot of time on their hands.) Having grown up Catholic, I understand what self-mortification is. I'm not a fan of pain for its own sake.

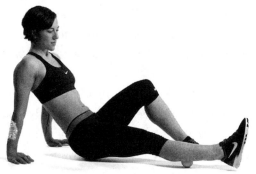

✳ Targeted Stretches

- Most experts recommend post-workout stretches because your muscles and connective tissues will be warmer and more pliable. But if you have a known problem area, it makes sense to work on it *before* lifting heavy things.
- Stretch muscles for 30 to 60 seconds, broken up however you like. Don't rest in between stretches for the same muscle; relax and then immediately repeat.

CALF ROLL

Roll over one calf at a time, using your nonworking leg as ballast to increase pressure.

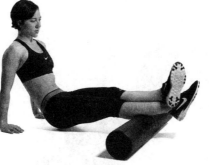

HAMSTRING ROLL

Same idea as the calf roll: Work one leg at a time, using the opposite leg to add pressure. Roll from the bottom of your knee to the gluteal crease, and back again, pulling and pushing yourself with your hands.

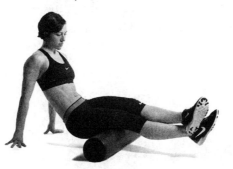

GLUTE ROLL

The fibers of the calves and hamstrings run parallel to your legs, but the fibers of your gluteus maximus run mostly perpendicular to them. So you want to roll east and west, rather than north and south. Work one glute at a time.

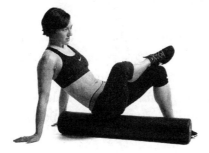

IT-BAND ROLL

Set the outside of your right hip on the roll, supporting your weight with your right hand and left foot on the floor, as shown. Work the outside of your right thigh, then switch sides and repeat.

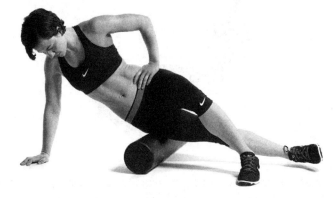

QUAD ROLL

Lie facedown for this one, with one thigh on the roll and the other leg on the floor. Pull yourself forward and back, using your arms and keeping your core braced.

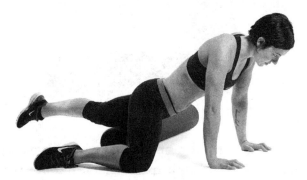

2. BREATHING RESET

Everything in fitness in cyclical. Take breathing, for example. When I started writing about exercise in the early 1990s, it was just understood that you needed to breathe in a specific sequence to make lifting safe and productive. We often included breathing instructions in workout articles. Eventually we came to realize that, because people already know how to breathe, we should focus on what they don't know how to do. Like, say, lifting.

But then, seemingly overnight, a new consensus formed around the idea that people *don't* know how to breathe. Friends and colleagues posted videos explaining the flaws in our inhalation and exhalation. They warned of the dire consequences of aberrant breathing and offered increasingly complex ways to fix the problem.

I mostly ignored it, as I ignore lots of things that seem overblown. But when I started using one of Alwyn's breathing drills at the beginning of each workout, I came around. It's like a warm-up for your respiratory system.

✴ Breathing Drills

The goal is always the same: pull air deep enough into your lungs to depress your diaphragm. Your belly will extend while your shoulders and ribs stay down. Then exhale. Alwyn and his trainers use several drills:

- Supine (faceup) on the floor, with legs bent or straight
- Supine, with hips and knees bent 90 degrees and feet flat against a wall as shown
- Prone (facedown), a drill called "crocodile breathing"
- In the child's pose from yoga: you're facedown, with your legs tucked beneath you and your chest on your thighs, arms extended, chin tucked

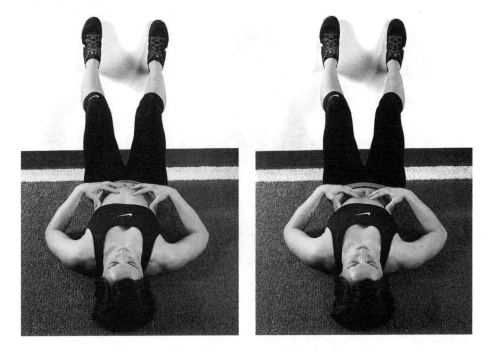

3. HIP MOBILITY

Successful lifting is possible only if you can keep your lower back and pelvis locked in a neutral position, with the lumbar spine in its natural arch. That's the safest and strongest position for supporting heavy weights. For that stability to occur, the joints above and below it need friction-free movement. So the first traditional exercise in RAMP is a stretch of the hip flexors, the strip of muscles on the front of your pelvis responsible for lifting your thighs closer to your torso.

✳ Hip-Flexor Stretch with Glute Activation

Rest your right knee on a pad, with your left knee bent and left foot flat on the floor in front of you. Set your knuckles on your glutes. Your torso is upright and perpendicular to the floor. Squeeze your right glute and shift your weight forward, feeling a stretch on the right side of your pelvis and down the front of your right thigh. Hold for 5 seconds. Relax your glute, reset your hips, and repeat. Do 6 reps/30 seconds per side.

Don't allow your lower back to hyperextend into a deeper arch. That shows your pelvis is tilting forward, which means you aren't actually stretching the hip flexors.

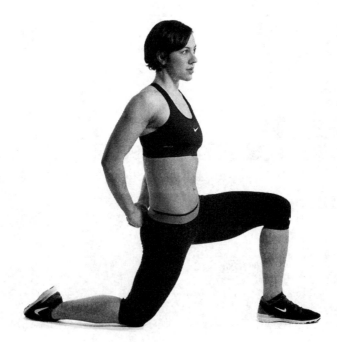

✳ Brettzel

This somewhat more advanced exercise, named after strength coach Brett Jones, stretches your rectus femoris (a hip-flexor muscle on the front of your thigh) along with your hips and middle back. The setup is a bit complicated:

- Lie on your left side, with your head resting on a pad or rolled-up towel that's 2 to 3 inches thick.
- Bend your right knee and raise your right thigh toward your chest, with the inside of your right knee and foot touching the floor. Hold it there with your left hand.
- Bend your left knee and grab your left shin with your right hand. Pull the foot up so your left heel is near your buttocks.
- Take a deep breath and try to align the left leg with your torso, keeping it firmly in place with your right hand.
- Now exhale and turn your head and shoulders to the right, while keeping your right knee in contact with the floor.
- Relax and reset. Do 3 or 4 reps.
- Switch sides and repeat.

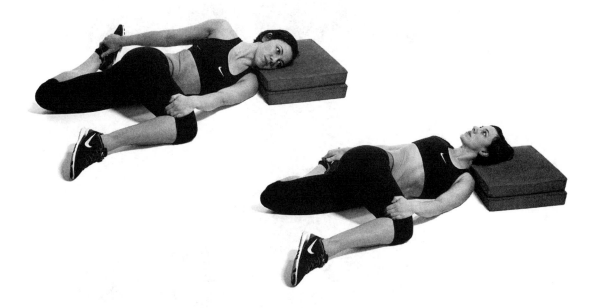

4. GLUTE ACTIVATION

The glutes are your body's strongest muscles, not to mention the most likely to draw third-party scrutiny (welcome or otherwise). They work with the hamstrings to straighten your hips when you're bent forward, which means they're the prime movers on deadlifts and also work hard on squats, lunges, step-ups, and swings. A glute-activation exercise makes sure they fire properly before you do any of the aforementioned exercises with heavy weights. You have lots of options.

✳ Hip Raise

This one's simple and easy: Lie on your back, knees bent, feet on the floor. Raise your hips until your body forms a straight line from chest to knees. Feel the squeeze in your glutes, but not in your lower back. Lower your hips near the floor, and repeat. Do 10 to 15.

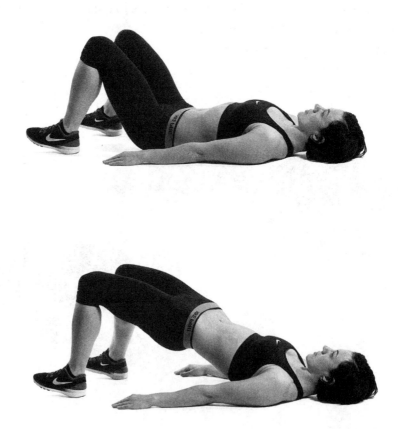

✳ Single-Leg Hip Raise

Same thing but with one leg extended. Start with the extended leg on the floor, and raise it along with your hips. At the top, it should be alongside the thigh of your working leg. Do 8 to 10 on each side.

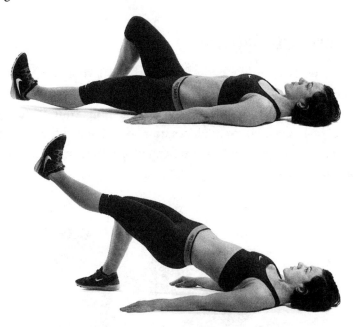

✳ Marching Hip Raise

Same setup as the other hip raises, only with your toes raised and your heels on the floor. Lift one leg as you raise your hips, keeping the knee bent. Lower it with your hips, then lift the opposite leg along with your hips. You'll probably feel this one more in your hamstrings and less in your glutes. Do 8 to 10 on each side.

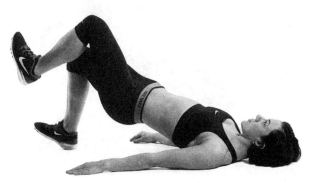

5. HIP AND UPPER-BACK MOBILITY

For your lumbar spine to stabilize successfully, its upstairs neighbor, the thoracic spine, has to move freely. Alwyn gives you two options here: You can either isolate this movement or combine it with a hip-mobility drill.

✳ Child's Pose with Rotation

Get into a modified child's pose: facedown, with your legs tucked beneath your chest, and your left forearm on the floor. Your right arm is bent, with your elbow next to your left arm and your fingers touching your temple just above your right ear. Now rotate your shoulders up and to the right, raising your right elbow as high as you can without turning your hips. Return to the starting position. Do 8 on each side.

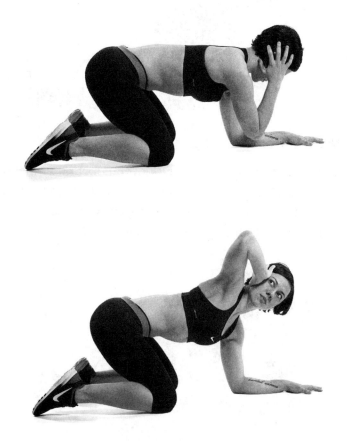

✳ Spider-Man Climb with Reach

Get into push-up position, with your hands directly below your shoulders. Step forward with your right foot until it's next to (or at least near) your right hand. Drop your hips until you feel a nice stretch in your lower abs and hip flexors. Lift your right hand and rotate your shoulders until both arms are perpendicular to the floor. Turn your head and follow your hand with your eyes. Now reverse the movement: Lower your hand to the floor, and step back to the starting position. Repeat with your left leg and arm. Alternate until you've done 5 to 6 on each side.

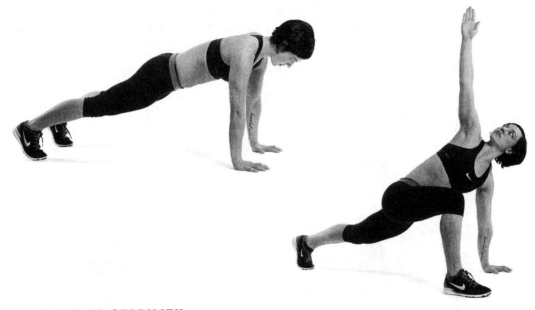

6. SCAPULAR STABILITY

Your scapulae, better known as your shoulder blades, are marvels of anatomical ingenuity. The trowel-shaped bones connect your upper arms to your collarbones, but otherwise float freely on the back of your rib cage. They move up and down and rotate in and out. Here's a partial list of muscles that attach to your scapulae:

- Biceps
- Triceps
- Trapezius (the diamond-shaped muscle in the middle of your back)
- Deltoids (shoulder muscles)
- All four parts of the rotator cuff

Like your hips, these unique and versatile joints need stability along with mobility. That is, they need to move freely when necessary, but also to control movement. You've already done one or two mobility exercises. Now it's time for one that focuses on stability.

✳ Wall Slide

Stand facing a wall, with the toes of your forward leg touching it. (It doesn't matter which leg is ahead of the other.) Rest your forearms against the wall so the tips of your fingers are level with your ears. Slide your arms up the wall as high as you can without losing contact with your forearms. Shrug your shoulders at the top to extend the range of motion. Do 8 to 10 reps.

Don't hyperextend your back. Stop if you feel your back sinking into a deeper arch.

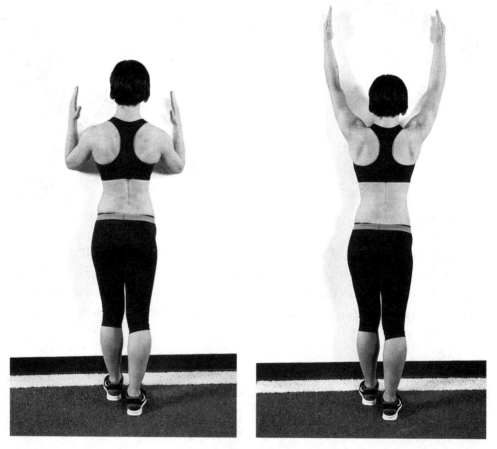

7. ANKLE MOBILITY

Now the focus moves from top to bottom. You can't move well without a full range of motion in your ankle joints.

✴ Single-Leg Calf Stretch from Push-Up Position

Set up in the push-up position. Rest the instep of your right foot behind your left ankle. Lift your hips into the pike position, with your upper torso and arms aligned at a 90-degree angle to your legs. Feel the stretch in the back of your left leg. Return to the push-up position and repeat. Do 3 to 5 with each leg.

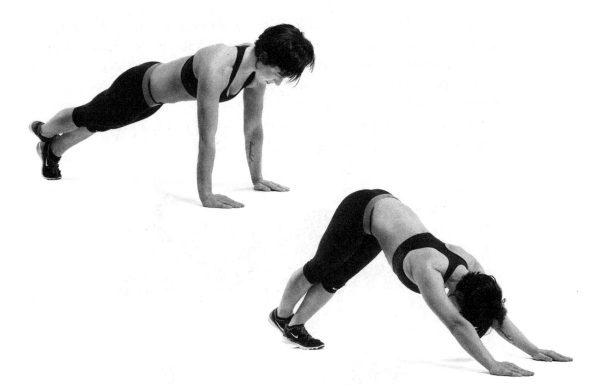

8. HIP STABILITY

The hip raises in the fourth category target stability for front-and-back movement—deadlifts, squats, and kettlebell swings. Now we shift to lateral movement, which is crucial in just about any sports context. If you can't move well to your left and right, you won't be very effective in basketball, soccer, softball, or tennis. In fact, it's hard to think of a sport where you *don't* use side-to-side movement.

"But what about running?" you say. "Or lifting? Isn't that all forward and back?"

Excellent questions, and they bring up the multiple roles played by your gluteus maximus. As my friend Bret Contreras likes to point out, the glutes exert a lot of force on the iliotibial band, the thick strip of connective tissue that runs along the outside of your leg from the hip, past your knee, to the tibia, the larger of your two lower-leg bones. The glutes thus help stabilize knee movement. I learned this lesson when I incorporated the following exercises and saw my chronic knee pain subside.

✳ Clamshell

Lie on your left side with your legs stacked on top of each other. You want your hips and torso to form a 135-degree angle, with your knees bent 90 degrees. Support your upper body on your left elbow. Lift your right knee as high as you can while keeping your left leg on the floor and your feet in contact with each other. Do 8 to 10 reps on each side.

Don't roll or shift your hips to extend the range of motion. If you don't feel this in your glutes, move your top leg forward just a bit.

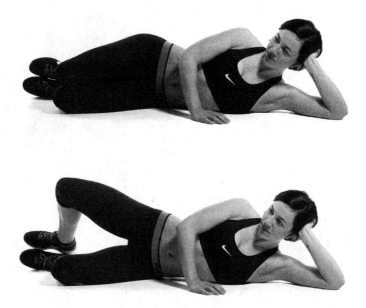

✳ **Walk with Mini Band**

I think this exercise, more than any other, gave me my knees back. You'll need a mini band, a cheap and useful piece of equipment I can't recommend highly enough. (You'll find more details in Appendix B.) Slide the band around your legs, just above your knees. Stand with your feet parallel and shoulder-width apart, and your body in an athletic posture. That is, your hips and knees are bent slightly, so you're ready to move in any direction. Take a long step to your left, keeping your feet parallel to each other. Bring your right leg up so your feet are once again shoulder-width apart, and immediately step again to your left. Do 8 to 10 reps to each side, and build up to 15 to 20. As your body gets used to the exercise, change things up by moving the band farther down your legs: below the knees, around the ankles, and eventually around your feet.

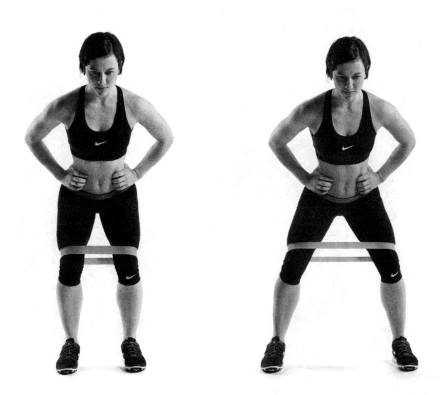

9. SQUAT

Now that we've activated the muscles that provide lateral stability, we're going to use them in the squat. The first option, the squat to stand, will be familiar to NROL readers; it's appeared in some form in four of the five books, starting with *NROL for Women*. It's a great mobility and flexibility exercise because the hamstrings get a good stretch in the top position. The second, the nose-to-wall squat, offers a test of balance as well as mobility.

✳ Squat to Stand

Stand with your feet parallel and shoulder-width apart. Bend forward at the hips and grab your toes (or your shins, if you can't reach that far). Pull yourself down into a squat, pushing your knees out with your arms. At the bottom, pull your shoulders down and back, which should push your chest forward. Now stand, feeling a nice stretch in your hamstrings as you straighten your legs. Do 8 to 10 reps, holding for a second or two at the bottom and top.

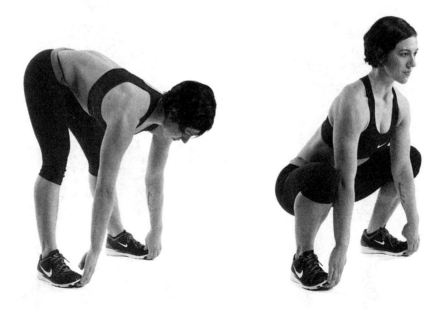

✳ **Nose-to-Wall Squat**

Stand facing a wall, with your toes and nose about 6 inches away from it. You want your feet about shoulder-width apart, with your toes pointed forward or angled out slightly. Extend your arms to the side so they're at a 45-degree angle to your torso, with your fingertips touching the wall. Push your hips back and descend into a squat, keeping your lower back and pelvis in the neutral position. Your form has to be perfect here; otherwise, your knees or nose will smack into the wall. Return to the starting position, keeping your fingertips on the wall throughout. Do 8 to 10 reps.

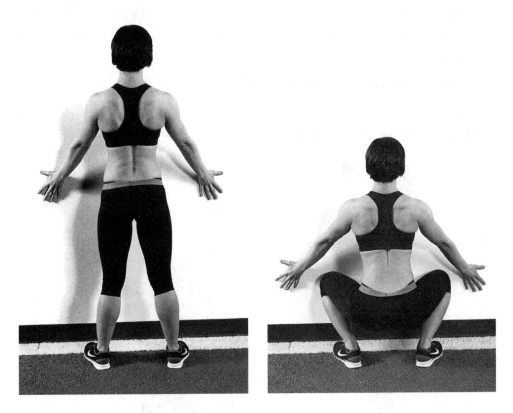

10. SINGLE-LEG BALANCE, HIP SEPARATION

Lots of goals here. *Single-leg balance* is a key element of Alwyn's programs. It activates big muscles, like those in your hips and thighs, along with smaller stabilizing muscles from your torso all the way down to your ankles and feet. *Hip separation* reflects the fact that in sports and life we rarely get to do things with our feet parallel to each other and our weight perfectly balanced. We need to be able to reach our end range of motion, as we do in a lunge, without damage to our muscles or connective tissues.

✳ Walking Knee Hug, Lunge, Reach

Stand with your feet about hip-width apart and some clear space in front of you. Lift your right knee, grab it with both hands, and pull it up to your chest. As you lower it, take a long step forward and drop into a lunge. Finish the movement by raising your arms overhead. Lower your arms, and as you come up out of the lunge, lift your left knee and pull it to your chest. Lunge forward with your left leg, and raise your arms. That's 1 repetition. Do 6 to 8.

"What If I Don't Have Enough Room?"

No problem. Do the knee hug, forward lunge, and reach. Then step back instead of forward, and repeat with the opposite leg.

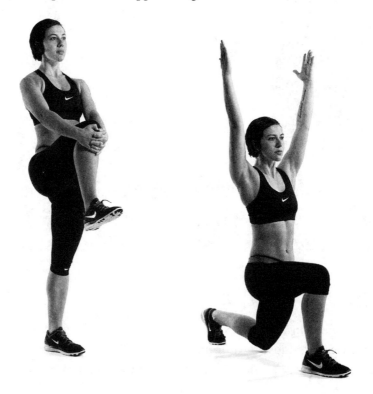

11. HIP SEPARATION, LATERAL MOVEMENT

Same idea as the single-leg balance and hip separation, but this time to the side.

✳ Walking Side Lunge

Stand with your feet hip-width apart. Take a long step to your left and descend into a side lunge. You should end up with your left knee bent about 90 degrees and right leg straight, with your body bent forward at the hips. As you rise, bring your right foot up so your feet are once again hip-width apart. Immediately lunge again with your left leg. Do 6 to 8, then reverse direction and repeat with your right leg.

Don't twist your shoulders or angle your feet out. You want to keep your shoulders square and your feet parallel to each other throughout the exercise.

"What If I Don't Have Enough Room?"

Lunge to one side, then lunge back in the opposite direction.

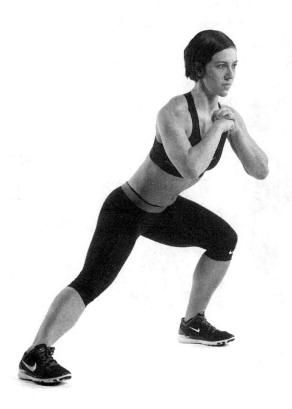

12. FORWARD OR LATERAL MOVEMENT, QUICK PACE

We finish in a flurry. If your body is ready to run—that is, to move both fast and well—you should be ready to lift. The simplest option is to jog 10 to 20 yards, and back again. So two short runs.

If you're feeling more energetic, you can do skips, side shuffles, carioca (a lateral-movement drill in which your hips and shoulders swivel with each step), or backward runs. That stuff is all fun when you belong to a gym where you have the space and the movements I just mentioned aren't unusual.

"What If I Don't Have the Space?"

Do 10 to 20 jumping jacks. Or, if you're more advanced, you can do mountain climbers, shown next.

✷ Mountain Climber

Get into push-up position. Bring one leg forward so your knee is beneath your chest, then pull it back and bring the other leg forward. Do it fast, so it feels like you're running in place, only with your hands on the floor. As noted, this is for the more advanced readers who have solid core stability and endurance. You don't want to exhaust those muscles before you even get to the core-training part of the program, which you'll see in the next chapter.

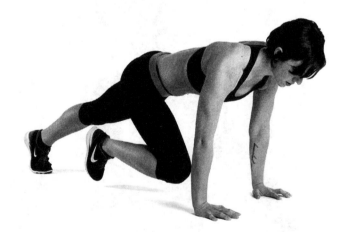

Core Training

The GOAL OF CORE TRAINING IS to improve stability. I offered a layman's definition of core stability in the last chapter: to keep your lower back and pelvis in a safe, neutral position. A more technical definition, one used by researchers, goes something like this:

The ability to control the position of your lumbar spine in order to produce, transfer, and manage force for sports and everyday activities.

Of those, *producing* force with your core muscles is the least important. Can you think of any task that requires you to do a sit-up with a weight that's heavier than what you could handle without any specific training? But *transferring* force is crucial to almost everything you do, in or out of the weight room. Picture yourself throwing a softball: Your hips and lower-body muscles generate power, which your core transfers through your shoulder and arm, culminating in the ball coming out of your hand many, many times faster than it would if you tried to throw without using those muscles.

It's also crucial for your core to *control* the force it transfers. As I noted in Chapter 11, the vertebrae of the lumbar spine have a very small range of motion. The core muscles have to transfer force in a way that prevents those vertebrae from moving beyond it. Imagine yourself driving a golf ball off a tee. The better you get, the harder you'll swing. The harder you swing, the easier it is for your lower back to bend or twist too far. Your health is contingent on your core stability improving along with your strength and skill.

Alwyn believes core stability is too important to leave for the end of the workout. By putting the core exercises in between the warm-up and the strength exercises, they play two roles: They're a continuation of RAMP because they activate the mid-body muscles. They're also the first *training* exercises, which means your goal is to improve performance from workout to workout.

Performance is exercise and context dependent.

If it's an isometric body-weight exercise, like a plank or side plank, you improve performance in three ways:

1. **Better form.** Don't be afraid to ask a trainer or knowledgeable workout partner to assess your technique. The position you hold should feel solid to you and look correct to an observer.
2. **Longer duration.** The workouts give you a maximum time to hold each static exercise and usually give you a choice of doing 1 or 2 sets. When you can hold the first set for the maximum, with good form, your next task is to reach maximum time on the second.
3. **More challenging variation.** Once you hit the maximum duration on 2 sets, you need to make the exercise itself more difficult. We'll show you options for each one.

If the exercise involves some kind of external resistance, you also have three ways to improve:

1. **Better form.** Doing the exercise well remains the top priority. This is traditionally a harder message to sell to men, who almost always want to use weights that are too heavy for their present skill level.
2. **More reps.** You want to reach the maximum recommended reps for every set before you increase the load.
3. **More weight.** This is traditionally a harder sell to women. When your form is good, and you can hit all your sets and reps, there's just one way to make prog-

ress: increase the load. If you don't, you're no longer training. You're just practicing something you've already trained your body to do. Embrace the opportunity.

PHASE ONE, STAGE 1

✴ Plank

WHERE IT IS: Phase One, Stage 1, Workout A

WHAT IT DOES: The plank is the most basic stabilization exercise, one that we classify as *anti-extension* because it trains your core muscles to hold your spine in the neutral position, preventing it from sinking into a deeper arch. Moreover, it develops endurance in the core muscles. A substantial body of research shows that endurance is the key to preventing or reducing back pain.

THE SETUP: All you need is a floor and a padded surface to protect your elbows.

HOW TO DO IT: Get into the plank position, with your weight resting on your forearms and toes and your body in a straight line from your neck through your ankles. Hold that position for up to 60 seconds.

PICTURE THIS: If you took a picture of yourself doing a plank, and then turned it 90 degrees, it should look like you were standing upright, only with your toes and forearms pushing into a wall. There should be no difference in your posture.

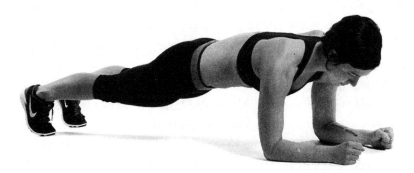

NOT READY FOR THIS ONE? Start with the *torso-elevated plank*. Rest your forearms on a bench, step, or padded box, which makes it a bit easier to hold the position. When you can hold an elevated plank for 30 seconds, try it again on the floor.

BADASS OPTIONS: If you can complete two 60-second holds, you have three ways to make the plank more challenging:

- Elevate your feet. This is the opposite of the torso-elevated plank, making it harder instead of easier.
- Reduce your base of support. Lift one arm or leg off the floor. For most of us, it'll be harder to do this on one side than the other. Start with the harder side, and then switch to the easier one halfway through the set.
- Extend the base of support. In the basic plank position, your arms are perpendicular to the floor. Move them forward, so they're diagonal to the floor. This changes your center of gravity and forces the core muscles to stabilize your body in an unfamiliar way.

✳ Bird Dog

WHERE IT IS: Phase One, Stage 1, Workout A

WHAT IT DOES: Walking upright was the first and most important evolutionary development on the path to becoming human. That's why our spinal column is narrowest at the top and thickest at the bottom; the thick part is what supports the weight of our torso and shoulders, in addition to whatever we might need to lift or carry. The bird dog, like the plank, plays a practical joke on our anatomy, turning the heaviest part of the spine from a support structure into a type of load that must be supported. These exercises do it in two different ways, with the plank primarily challenging the muscles on the front of the abdomen and the bird dog targeting the ones in the lower back.

THE SETUP: All you need is a floor and a padded surface to protect your elbows.

HOW TO DO IT: Start on your hands and knees. Lift your left arm and right leg and push them straight out from your shoulders and hips, as if you're encountering some kind of resistance. Stop when they're parallel to your torso. Hold that position for up to 15 seconds. Now pull them back, once again moving as if something stronger than gravity were holding them back. Repeat with your right arm and left leg. You want to do a total of 4 extensions with each arm and leg, which will take up to 2 minutes if you hold each extension for the full 15 seconds.

PICTURE THIS: Imagine that you're Superman flying, only without the cape, the tights, and the vaguely superior smirk on your face. Your body forms a straight line from your neck to your tailbone, and your hips and shoulders remain parallel to the floor at all times—no twisting or shifting. Most important of all: *There should be no additional arching of your back.*

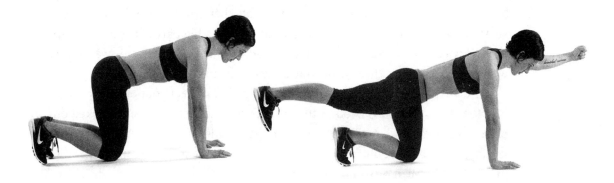

NOT READY FOR THIS ONE? If you can't hold for 15 seconds, or even 5 seconds, simply move your arms and legs in and out at the most deliberate pace you can manage.

BADASS OPTION: If you can complete the full 2-minute sequence with good form, you've earned the right to do a variation that's so much harder you'll wish you could go back to the bird dog: *push-up hold with arm and leg extended.* Start in the push-up position, and raise your right arm and left leg. Hold for up to 15 seconds, then switch sides and repeat. If you can do *that* for the full 2 minutes, go write your own workout books, because you're much better at this than I'll ever be.

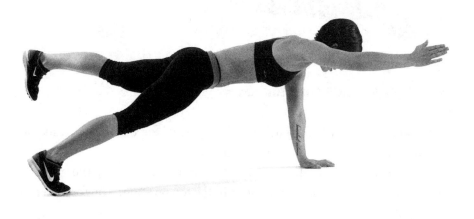

✳ Side Plank

WHERE IT IS: Phase One, Stage 1, Workout B

WHAT IT DOES: We classify the side plank as an *anti-lateral-flexion* exercise, because it trains your torso to remain upright when lifting an unbalanced load. If you have small children, lifting unbalanced loads is a big part of the job description (as discussed in Chapter 1). But even if you don't, this is a solid training exercise that works the muscles on the side of your body closest to the floor.

THE SETUP: All you need is a floor and a pad to protect your elbow.

HOW TO DO IT: Lie on your left side, with your legs straight and stacked on top of each other. Your weight is supported on the outside edge of your left foot and your left forearm. Your left upper arm is directly below your shoulder and perpendicular to the floor. You can rest your right hand on your right hip or your left shoulder. Lift your hips so you form a straight line from your nose through your belly button. Hold for 30 seconds, switch sides, and repeat.

PICTURE THIS: Ideally, as with the plank, a photo of you in a side plank could be turned to make it look like you were standing upright, with your left arm raised for no apparent reason.

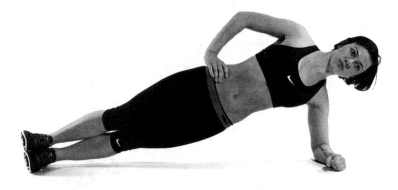

NOT READY FOR THIS ONE? You have a couple of options:

- Do a *modified side plank*, with your knees bent, so your weight rests on your forearm and the outside of your bottom knee.
- Do *hip raises*, starting with your hips on the floor and lifting them to the side-plank position. Hold for a few seconds in the top position. Aim for 30 seconds of work per side.

BADASS OPTIONS: There are a couple of basic ways to make the side plank more challenging:

- Elevate your feet.
- Reduce your base of support by lifting your top leg while keeping both legs straight.

✳ Cable Half-Kneeling Antirotation Press

WHERE IT IS: Phase One, Stage 1, Workout B

WHAT IT DOES: The function is in the name: It trains your body to resist spinal rotation.

THE SETUP: Attach a D-shaped handle to the cable pulley, and set it to mid-thigh height. (You can also do this and other cable exercises with a band, attaching it to something sturdy like a squat rack.) Because you'll be kneeling, you want to make sure to protect your knee.

HOW TO DO IT: Grab the handle with both hands and kneel sideways to the cable machine, with the knee closest to the machine on the floor. Pull the handle to your chest as you straighten your torso, with your shoulders square. Now press the weight straight out from your chest, and hold it there for 10 seconds. Pull it back under full

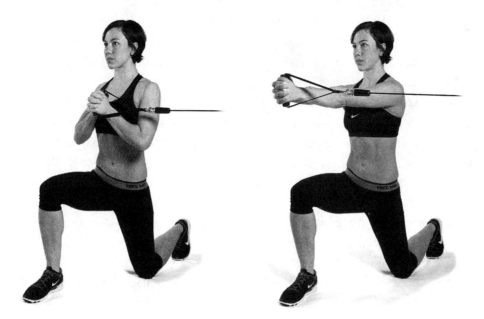

control, hold at your chest for 1 second, and then press it out again. Do 3 reps, holding each for 10 seconds with your arms fully extended. Switch sides and repeat.

KEY POINT: Make sure you're far enough from the weight stack (or the attachment point for your band) that you have tension in the cable or band from start to finish.

PICTURE THIS: The object is to create the illusion that you're doing a chest press, even though the resistance is coming from the side, rather than the front. Keep your torso upright and your shoulders square.

BADASS OPTIONS: There really aren't any. If you struggle, drop the weight until you can do the press as described. And if you're a badass, increase the weight until you feel challenged. But keep in mind that form matters more than weight. Most people I've observed over the years will hike up one shoulder and/or bend slightly in one direction or the other—understabilizing if they lean toward the machine; overcompensating for the resistance if they lean away from it.

PHASE ONE, STAGE 2

✳ Plank with Pulldown

WHERE IT IS: Phase One, Stage 2, Workout A

WHAT IT DOES: If you're like me, this exercise will kind of piss you off. That's because it's hard and it exposes your weaknesses. It's an anti-extension, *dynamic-stability* exercise (if you're not into that whole brevity thing). The "dynamic" part comes from the fact you're generating force with one arm while using the other three limbs to stabilize your body in the plank position.

WHAT MAKES IT SO CHALLENGING: Your lats are key stabilizing muscles. The upper fibers attach to your thoracic vertebrae, the lower ones attach to the top of your pelvis, and the ones in between merge with your thoracolumbar fascia, a thick network of connective tissue that extends all the way to your tailbone. When your lats are contracted, they naturally support the arch in your lower back. But when you extend your arm, you lose that support and have to make up with it with other stabilizing muscles. Put another way, you're asking your lats to do two things at once: act as a prime mover for an exercise while also acting as a key stabilizer. Whatever weight you use, it'll feel like a lot more.

THE SETUP: Attach a D-shaped handle to a cable pulley set in the lowest position. (You can also use a band.) Position yourself in a plank, facing the weight stack. You probably want to move your feet apart to provide a wider base.

HOW TO DO IT: Grab the handle with your right hand. Make sure there's tension in the cable or band with your arm fully extended. (If not, scoot back until there is.) Pull the handle to the top of your chest, or as close as you can get. Pause, and return to the starting position. Do 12 reps, then switch sides and repeat.

PICTURE THIS: It's probably best if you don't picture *anything*; just try to keep your entire body parallel to the floor throughout the exercise. One of the biggest challenges is keeping your neck aligned with your torso. Your natural inclination is to raise your head so you can see the weight as you move it.

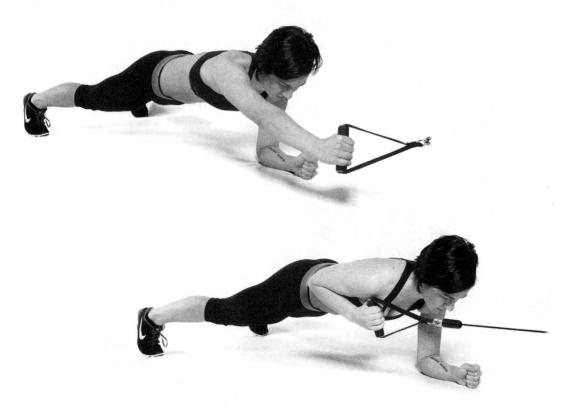

✳ Side Plank with Row

WHERE IT IS: Phase One, Stage 2, Workout B

WHAT IT DOES: It does double-duty as an anti-lateral-flexion and antirotation exercise, and unlike the plank with pulldown, it's kind of fun to do. But just because it's not annoying doesn't mean it's not challenging. You'll have to work hard to keep your body in the correct position.

THE SETUP: Attach a D-shaped handle to a cable pulley in the lowest position. (You can also use a band.) Face the machine as you get into side-plank position, with your top shoulder even with the cable.

HOW TO DO IT: Grab the handle with your top hand. Make sure there's tension in the cable, and hold it with your palm toward the floor. Set your body in a straight line from your nose to your belly button. Pull the handle to the top of your rib cage, on whatever line allows you to avoid hitting your breast. Return to the starting position under complete control. Do 12 reps, then switch sides and repeat.

PICTURE THIS: Imagine that there's a wall behind you, keeping you from leaning back. The key to the antirotation effect of the exercise is to keep your body in a plane that's perpendicular to the floor.

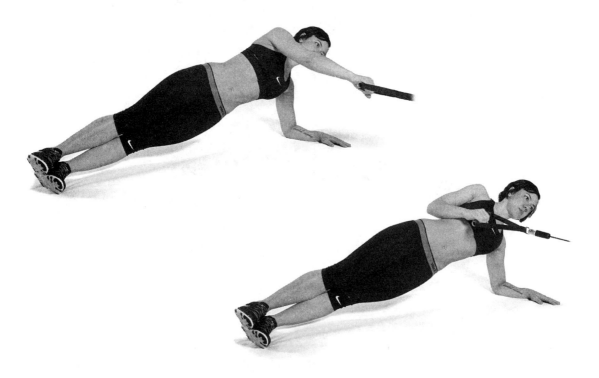

PHASE ONE, STAGE 3

✳ Valslide Push-Away

WHERE IT IS: Phase One, Stage 3, Workout A

WHAT IT DOES: Another anti-extension exercise, but this time you're pushing one arm away from your center of gravity, rather than pulling it toward you, as you did in the plank with pulldown. This type of exercise—similar to the rollouts and fallouts you'll find later in the program—has been shown to work the rectus abdominis, the "six-pack" muscle, harder than crunches and sit-ups.

THE SETUP: You'll need a pair of Valslides, or another type of sliding disc. (Appendix B includes multiple options, including a towel if you're on a wood or tile floor.) Set one under each hand and get into push-up position: arms straight and directly under your shoulders, feet about hip-width apart, body in a straight line from neck to ankles.

HOW TO DO IT: Slide your right hand forward as far as you can, keeping your lower back in the neutral position and both arms straight. Pull it back, and slide your left hand forward. That's 2 reps; shoot for 12 per set.

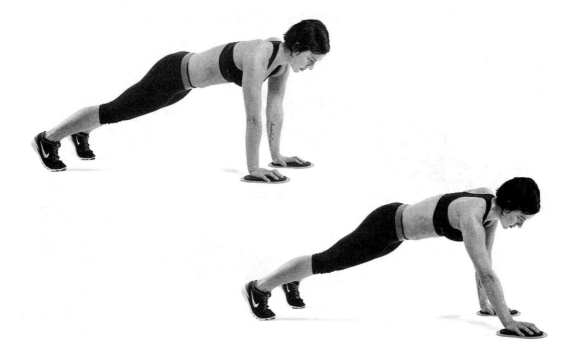

RANGE OF MOTION: When we wrote *NROL for Abs*, I got down on the floor and measured the distance I could slide forward before I had to bend my arms. It was 15 inches. While writing this book, five years later, it was more like 20 inches. I don't think my arms got longer, and I can't think of any reason why my performance would improve so dramatically. If there's a lesson here, it's that range of motion doesn't matter as much as effort. As long as you feel a challenge to your abdominal muscles and no strain to your lower back, you're doing it right.

BADASS OPTION: We've included the push-away in several books, and in the process we unintentionally gave readers two different ways to count reps. The correct way is what you see here: Do half the reps with each arm. But in a couple of books we said to do all the reps with each arm. That's how I did them this time around: 12 push-aways with each arm, each set. I didn't understand why it was so brutal until I realized I was counting wrong. So that's your badass challenge: Count wrong, and do more than the workout requires.

✳ Alternating Side Plank

WHERE IT IS: Phase One, Stage 3, Workout B

WHAT IT DOES: This adds a balance challenge to the basic plank and side plank, along with a very slight conditioning challenge, in that you may find yourself a little winded the first time you try it.

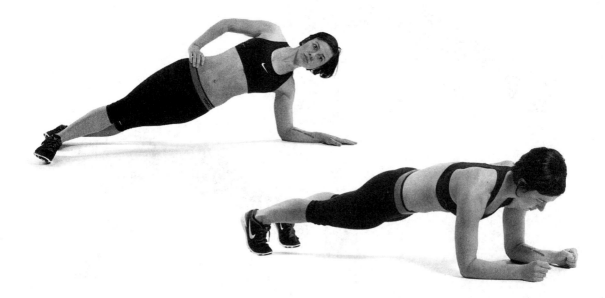

THE SETUP: Just your standard plank position, with some kind of padding to protect your elbows.

HOW TO DO IT: From the plank position, rotate to your right, into the side-plank position. Hold that position for 3 seconds. Return to the plank position. Rotate to your left and again hold for 3 seconds. Continue alternating until you've done 5 reps on each side.

BADASS OPTION: The side plank with oblique crunch is a different exercise but a fun way to mix things up. Start in the side-plank position, only with your bottom arm straight. Raise your top knee and bring your top elbow down to meet it. Rotate and repeat on the opposite side.

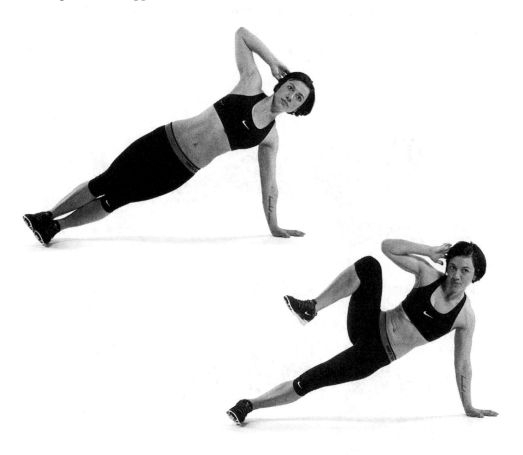

PHASE TWO, STAGE 4

✴ Suspended Plank

WHERE IT IS: Phase Two, Stage 4, Workout A

WHAT IT DOES: With your feet suspended above the floor, you're introducing an element of instability to the plank. It should be a simple progression, but whatever imbalances you have in your support structure will be exposed here. I'm humbled every time I reintroduce it to my workouts.

THE SETUP: You'll need a suspension system, like the TRX shown here. (You'll find some options in Appendix B.) You also want some serious padding to protect your elbows.

HOW TO DO IT: Set your feet in the stirrups, get into the plank position, and hold for up to 60 seconds.

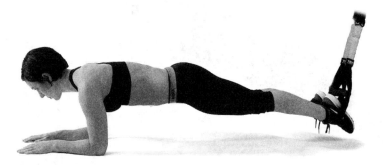

NO SUSPENSION SYSTEM? Do a *push-up hold* with your feet on a Swiss ball.

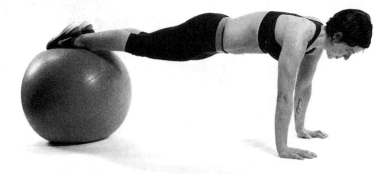

BADASS OPTIONS: If you can do 2 sets, 60 seconds each, you have two ways to make it more challenging:

- Raise the straps, so your feet are higher.
- Put one foot in the straps and keep the other next to it without support.

✳ Half-Kneeling Cable Chop

WHERE IT IS: Phase Two, Stage 4, Workout A

WHAT IT DOES: This antirotation exercise actually involves some rotation, in that your arms travel in a high-to-low diagonal path across your torso. But your hips and shoulders remain in place, which means all the movement involves your torso muscles.

THE SETUP: Attach a rope to the high cable pulley, and slide the ring, which is normally in the middle of the rope, to the end closest to the machine. Make sure you have a pad for your knee.

HOW TO DO IT: Grab the rope overhand, with your hands as far apart as possible (probably 24 inches). Kneel sideways to the machine, with the closest leg up and the other down. Straighten your torso. Pull the rope down and across your torso. The

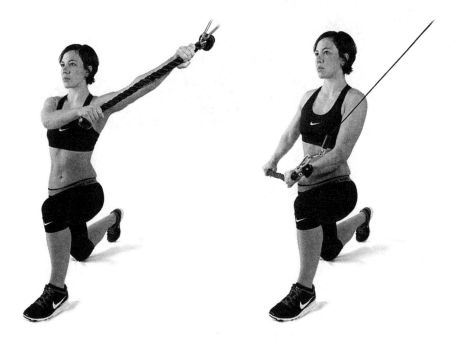

hand closest to the cable machine should end up in front of your outside hip, while your hips and shoulders remain in place. Do 10 reps, switch sides, and repeat.

✳ Suspended Side Plank

WHERE IT IS: Phase Two, Stage 4, Workout B

WHAT IT DOES: As with the suspended plank, you're working with an unstable base. Whatever weaknesses you have will be exposed.

THE SETUP: You'll need a suspension system, like the TRX shown here. (You'll find some options in Appendix B.) You also want some serious padding to protect your elbows.

HOW TO DO IT: Set your feet in the stirrups. Turn sideways as you get into position, with your feet stacked on top of each other. Rest your bottom elbow on the pad, lift your hips, and straighten your body. Hold for up to 60 seconds per side. Most of us will do 2 sets of 30 seconds per side. But if you can hold for 60 seconds per side on the first set, there's no need to do another.

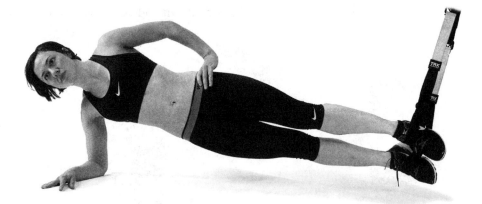

✳ Half-Kneeling Cable Lift

WHERE IT IS: Phase Two, Stage 4, Workout B

WHAT IT DOES: Same as the half-kneeling cable chop, but I find the lift harder to do. Even with less weight, my grunt-to-rep ratio goes up substantially.

THE SETUP: Attach a rope to the low cable pulley, and slide the ring to the end of the rope.

HOW TO DO IT: Grab the rope overhand, with your hands as far apart as possible, and kneel sideways to the machine, with the closest knee on the floor and the other one up. Straighten your body. Pull the rope up and across your torso. The hand closest to the cable machine should end up in front of your outside shoulder, while your hips and shoulders remain in place. Do 10 reps, switch sides, and repeat.

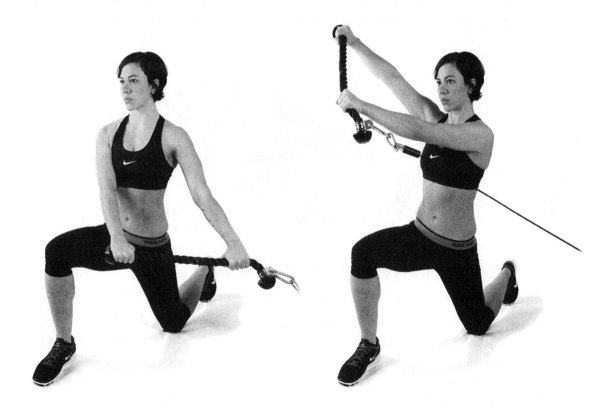

PHASE TWO, STAGE 5

✳ Valslide Mountain Climber

WHERE IT IS: Phase Two, Stage 5, Workout A

WHAT IT DOES: Mountain climbers work your hip flexors, the muscles that lift your thighs up in front of you. But the real value of the exercise comes from the work the rest of your core muscles do to provide stability. Where you feel it most probably depends on where you're most vulnerable. For me, that's my lower abdomen. For you, it might be the lower back, middle back, or even the upper back. All those muscles have to work hard to keep your torso stable while you move your legs up and down.

THE SETUP: You just need a pair of sliding discs.

HOW TO DO IT: Get into the push-up position with the balls of your feet on the discs. From there, it's like you're running. As you pull one leg up toward your chest, you push the other one back. Do as many as you can, rest, and repeat.

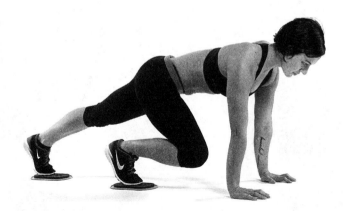

✳ Suspended Fallout or Rollout Variation

WHERE IT IS: Phase Two, Stage 5, Workout B

WHAT IT DOES: Like the push-away in Phase One, Stage 3, the fallout is an anti-extension exercise that offers a tough challenge to your core, especially the rectus abdominis.

THE SETUP: If you've never done this exercise before, you probably want to start with the handles of the suspension system at about mid-thigh height, or perhaps a little higher. If it's too easy, you can always set them lower for the next set, and for subsequent workouts.

HOW TO DO IT: Grab the handles and set up in push-up position, with your toes on the floor, your body angled forward, and your arms straight and perpendicular to your torso. Fall forward, slowly and under full control, as you extend your arms out in front of you. Go as low as you can while keeping your body straight, with at most a slight bend in your hips. Pull back to the starting position and repeat.

Don't sacrifice form to get a bigger range of motion. On YouTube, everyone finishes the exercise fully extended, like a superhero. In real life, you rarely see anyone with that range of motion.

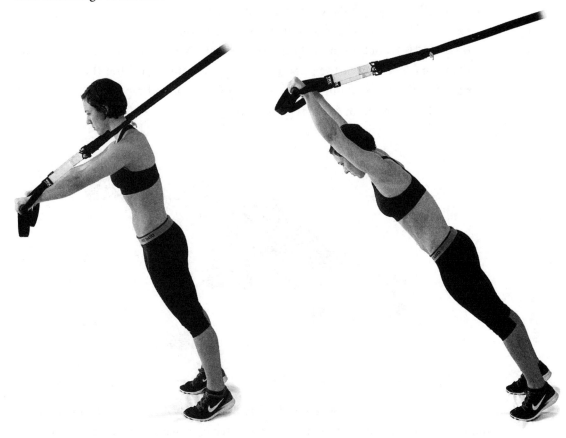

NOT READY FOR THIS ONE? Try the *Swiss-ball rollout*: Get into plank position with your forearms on the ball, toes on the floor, and feet spread wide apart for stability. Set your body in two straight lines: from your neck to your hips, and from your hips to your ankles, with just a slight forward bend in your hips. Roll the ball forward, straightening your arms and lowering your torso as far as you can while keeping your back in the neutral position. Roll back and repeat.

PHASE TWO, STAGE 6

✳ Valslide Spider-Man Push-Away

WHERE IT IS: Phase Two, Stage 6, Workout A

WHAT IT DOES: It combines two tough movements: the push-away, which you did in Phase One, Stage 3, and the Spider-Man, which is similar to a mountain climber, only with your leg to the side instead of beneath you. The combination tests your strength, stability, balance, and coordination.

THE SETUP: You just need sliding discs and a floor.

HOW TO DO IT: Set up in push-up position, with your hands on the discs. Slide your left hand out, and at the same time lift your right leg off the floor and raise your knee to your side. Return to the starting position, and repeat with your right arm and left leg. Shoot for 6 to 8 reps per side.

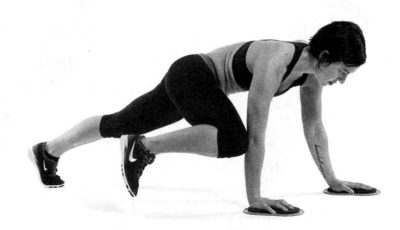

NOT READY FOR THIS ONE? Join the club! I got only 4 reps per side my first try, and I'd be surprised if I'm the only one who struggles with it. You can do the exercise without the slides: From the push-up position, move your right hand forward a few inches, then raise your left knee to your side. Return to the starting position, and repeat with the other arm and leg. Go for 6 to 8 reps per side.

✳ Split-Stance Cable Chop

WHERE IT IS: Phase Two, Stage 6, Workout A

WHAT IT DOES: It's the same as the half-kneeling cable chop, only without a knee on the floor to anchor your position.

THE SETUP: Attach a rope to the high cable pulley, and slide the ring to the end closest to the machine.

HOW TO DO IT: Grab the rope overhand, with your hands as far apart as possible. Stand sideways to the machine, with the closest leg forward and your foot flat on the floor. Your rear leg is back, with your weight on the ball of the foot. Stand up straight. Pull the rope down and across your torso. The hand closest to the cable machine should end up in front of your outside hip, while your hips and shoulders remain in place. Do 12 reps, switch sides, and repeat.

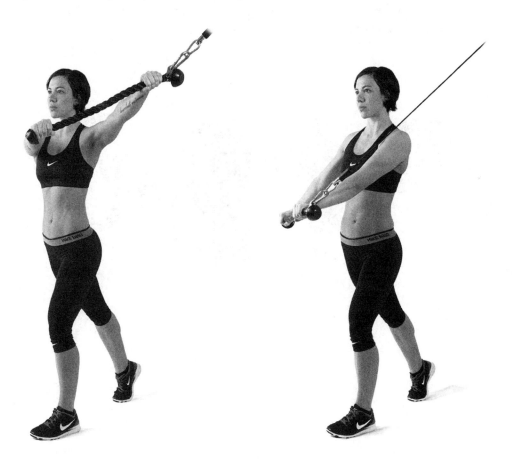

✳ Suspended Jackknife

WHERE IT IS: Phase Two, Stage 6, Workout B

WHAT IT DOES: Like the mountain climber, the jackknife is a hip-flexion exercise. Interestingly, in a study of core exercises using an unstable surface (a Swiss ball), this one showed some of the highest activity recorded for the external obliques, the muscles on the sides of your waist.

THE SETUP: Set the stirrups of the suspension system to about mid-calf height (8 to 12 inches above the floor).

HOW TO DO IT: Get into push-up position with your feet in the stirrups. Set your body in a straight line from neck to ankles. Pull your knees toward your chest, keeping your back flat. Return to the starting position and repeat. Do 10 reps.

Don't tuck your tailbone at the end. Your lower back and pelvis must remain in the neutral position, even if you sacrifice a few inches of your range of motion.

NO SUSPENSION SYSTEM? Do the same exercise on a Swiss ball.

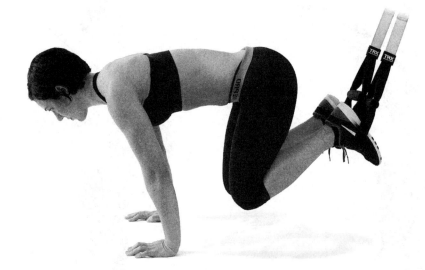

✳ Split-Stance Cable Lift

WHERE IT IS: Phase Two, Stage 6, Workout B

WHAT IT DOES: It's the same as the half-kneeling cable lift, only without a knee on the floor.

THE SETUP: Attach a rope to the low cable pulley, and slide the ring to the end closest to the machine.

HOW TO DO IT: Grab the rope overhand, with your hands as far apart as possible. Stand sideways to the machine, with the closest leg back, your weight on the ball of the foot, and your other leg forward. That foot is flat on the floor. Stand up straight. Pull the rope up and across your torso. The hand closest to the cable machine should end up in front of your outside shoulder, while your hips and shoulders remain in place. Do 10 reps, switch sides, and repeat.

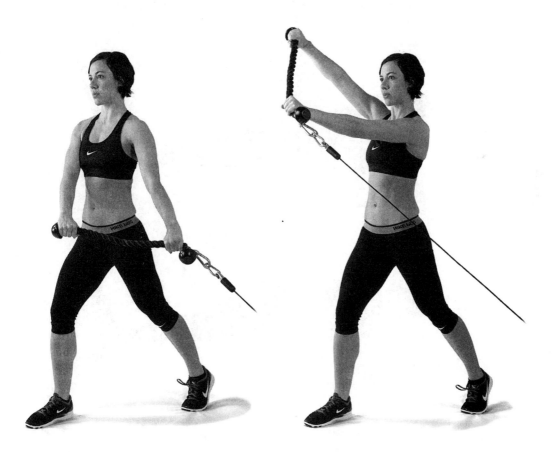

PHASE THREE, STAGE 7

✴ Suspended Body Saw

WHERE IT IS: Phase Three, Stage 7, Workout A

WHAT IT DOES: It's like a rollout, only with muscle activation in both directions—pushing back and pulling forward. A study in the *Journal of Sports Sciences* found that it lit up abdominal muscles with minimal strain on the spine. It's also probably the best exercise in Alwyn's program for the serratus anterior, a fingerlike set of muscles on the sides of your rib cage.

THE SETUP: Set the stirrups of the suspension system to about mid-calf height. Make sure you have a pad to protect your elbows.

HOW TO DO IT: Set your feet in the stirrups and get into plank position with your forearms on the pad. Push back as far as you can while keeping your back in the neutral position. Then pull forward as far as you can. Do 8 to 12 reps.

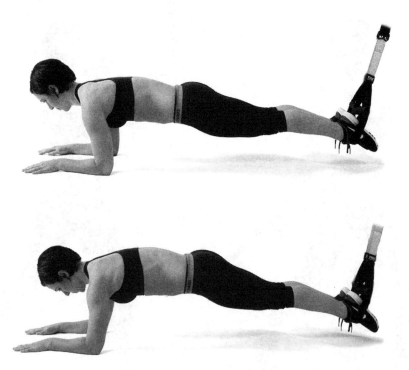

NO SUSPENSION SYSTEM? You can do the body saw with your feet on sliding discs. Or if you don't have those either, you can try it on a Swiss ball. Start in the push-up position with your lower legs on the ball. Push back, then pull forward. Do this slowly; if you're impatient, your momentum combined with the ball's buoyancy will make it both easy and sloppy.

BADASS OPTIONS: As you get stronger, the exercise naturally becomes more challenging because you'll increase your range of motion.

✴ Suspended Pike

WHERE IT IS: Phase Three, Stage 7, Workout B

WHAT IT DOES: In a study in the *Journal of Sports Sciences*, mentioned a moment ago, the pike was the only exercise that registered higher activation of the obliques than the jackknife. It was also shown to be one of the two best for overall muscle recruitment, along with the rollout. Fair warning: The volunteers in the study rated it the hardest one to perform.

THE SETUP: Set the stirrups of the suspension system to about mid-calf height.

HOW TO DO IT: Put your feet in the stirrups and get into push-up position. Keeping your arms and legs straight and back flat, raise your hips up toward the ceiling. Done with perfect form, your torso and arms will finish perpendicular to the floor, while your legs form a 45-degree angle with your torso. Do 8 to 12 reps.

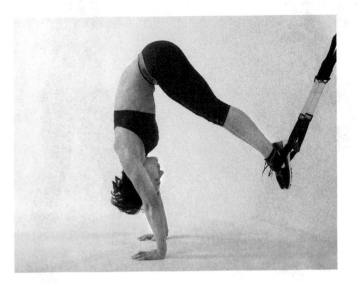

✳ Standing Antirotation Press + Overhead Raise

WHERE IT IS: Phase Three, Stage 7, Workout C

WHAT IT DOES: As you can guess from its title, this exercise does a lot of things. Like the antirotation press way back in Phase One, Stage 1, it trains your body to resist forces that would otherwise cause your back to bend and twist. But that earlier exercise had you work from a more stable, balanced position. By pressing overhead, instead of straight out, you're moving the resistance as far as possible from your center of gravity.

THE SETUP: Attach a D-shaped handle to a cable pulley that's set at mid-chest height.

HOW TO DO IT: Take the handle with both hands, stand sideways to the machine with your legs shoulder-width apart, and pull the handle to your chest. Push it out and up over your head, keeping your shoulders and hips square. Lower it to your chest and repeat. Do 8 to 12 reps.

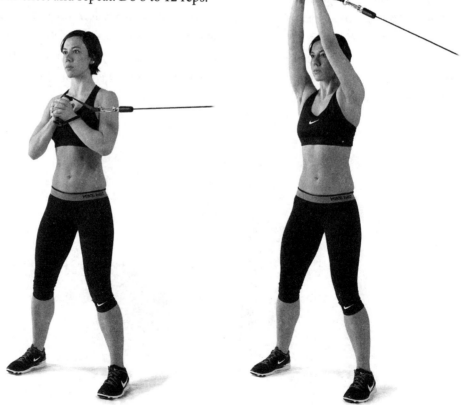

PHASE THREE, STAGE 8

✳ Ab-Wheel Rollout

WHERE IT IS: Phase Three, Stage 8, Workout A

WHAT IT DOES: It's the best-known rollout exercise (other than perhaps the old-school barbell rollout, which it mostly replaced) and does all the same things as the similar exercises you've already tried: Valslide push-away, suspended fallout, and body saw. Because the wheel is easier to control than the other devices, you'll feel it more directly in your midsection.

THE SETUP: All you need is an ab wheel—a lawnmower wheel with handles on the sides—and a pad for your knees. You can get a wheel online for $10 or less. (The one used in our photos is a bigger, more expensive version, as explained in Appendix B.)

HOW TO DO IT: Kneel on the pad and grab the handles. Straighten your body so there's a straight line from your neck to your pelvis. Push the wheel forward until you feel some tension on your core; at that point your body will form a 45-degree angle to the floor, while your arms form a 90-degree angle to your torso and thighs. Lean forward from the knees as you roll the wheel out. Go as far as you can, stopping if you feel any shift in your lower back. Pull back to the starting position. Do 8 to 10 reps.

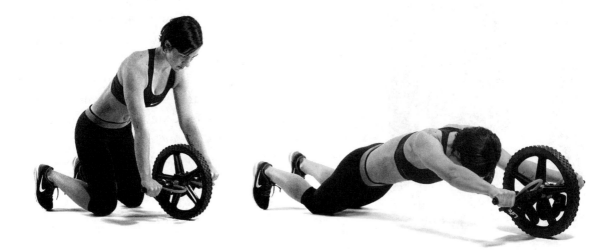

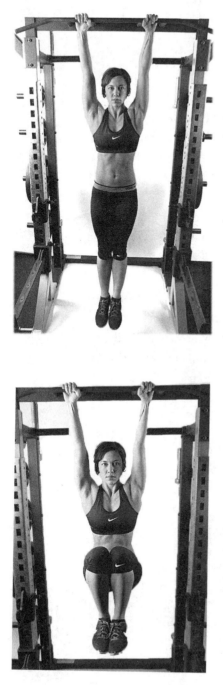

NOT READY FOR THIS ONE? Even for an advanced lifter, this exercise can be problematic. If you have any history of abdominal-muscle injury, such as diastasis recti from a pregnancy, you probably want to avoid it. (I say this as an involuntary member of the herniated-American community.) The *Journal of Sports Sciences* study mentioned earlier showed the *hand walkout* is a good alternative, challenging your rectus abdominis as well as your serratus. Execution is simple: Get into the push-up position and walk your hands out as far as you can while keeping your back in the neutral position. Pause, and then walk them back.

✷ Hanging Knee Raise

WHERE IT IS: Phase Three, Stage 8, Workout B

WHAT IT DOES: The hanging leg raise, with straight legs, is among the most badass exercises you can do. Not only does it force the abdominal muscles to work as hard as possible, it activates lots of other muscles as well, including the pectorals, lats, and quadriceps. But with those benefits comes risk, as compression forces on the spine reach potentially dangerous levels. The hanging knee raise, by contrast, puts far less pressure on the back, while still providing a challenge to your abdominal muscles.

THE SETUP: You just need a chin-up bar.

HOW TO DO IT: Grab the bar overhand, with your hands about shoulder-width apart. Bend your knees as you raise your thighs to your chest, while keeping your arms straight. Lower your legs and repeat. Do 8 to 10 reps.

✳ Cable Horizontal Chop

WHERE IT IS: Phase Three, Stage 8, Workout C

WHAT IT DOES: Unlike the diagonal chops and lifts you've done throughout the program, this one goes straight across. I'm a big fan of this exercise; you can use more weight than on the aforementioned exercises and feel it more directly in your abdominals. With heavier weights you'll also get some work for your upper-torso muscles.

THE SETUP: Attach a D-shaped handle to the cable pulley and set it to about mid-chest height.

HOW TO DO IT: Take the handle with both hands and stand sideways to the machine, your feet parallel to each other and spread wide to give you a solid base. Straighten your arms so the handle is in front of your chest. Let the cable pull your arms toward the machine as far as possible while keeping your arms straight and your shoulders and hips square. That's your starting position. Pull as far away from the machine as you can without turning your shoulders or hips. That's 1 rep. Do 10, switch sides, and repeat.

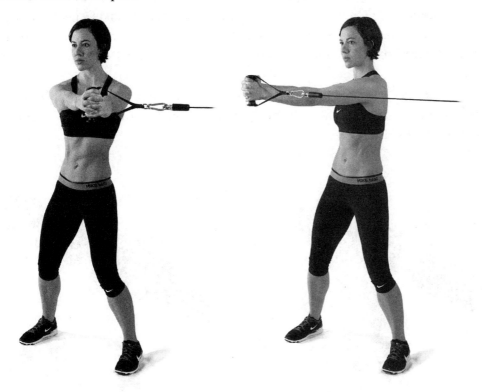

PHASE THREE, STAGE 9

✳ Dumbbell Plank Row

WHERE IT IS: Phase Three, Stage 9, Workout A

WHAT IT DOES: By itself, the basic push-up is a pretty good core exercise. Add any additional challenge, and it becomes a *great* one. (More on that in Chapter 14.) This exercise, also known as the renegade row, is a perfect example. With each row, you reduce your base of support. Naturally, that sends an SOS to all the muscles in your torso and hips, forcing them to figure out a stabilizing strategy while simultaneously activating upper-back and shoulder muscles to lift the dumbbell with the arm that's no longer providing support. It doesn't matter how heavy the weight is. The inefficiency of the movement activates more muscles, and offers a greater systemic challenge to your body than you would get from doing a row with heavier weight in a more stable position.

THE SETUP: Grab a pair of light dumbbells and set them on the floor.

HOW TO DO IT: Get into push-up position with your hands on the dumbbells. You probably want to do this with your hands closer together and feet wider apart. Set your body in a straight line. Pull the dumbbell in your right hand to the right side of your torso. Lower it to the floor. Repeat with your left. Do 8 to 10 with each arm.

NOT READY FOR THIS ONE? It's a bit easier to work one side at a time, with your nonworking hand on the floor. If that's still too much, do the exercise as described, only without weights.

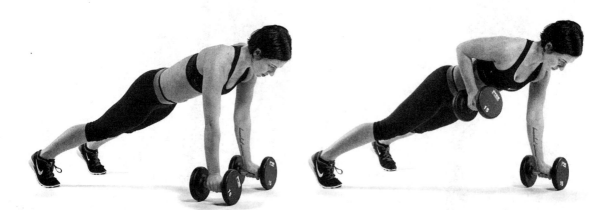

✳ **Windmill**

WHERE IT IS: Phase Three, Stage 9, Workout B

WHAT IT DOES: This adaptation of an old-time strongman exercise offers a unique set of challenges. It requires mobility in your hips and hamstrings, while developing strength and stability in your upper back and shoulders.

THE SETUP: You just need a light kettlebell. You can also use a dumbbell, although it'll be a little harder to balance.

HOW TO DO IT: Grab the kettlebell with your right hand and raise it straight over your right shoulder. Set your feet shoulder-width apart, and rotate them 45 degrees to your left. Turn your head so your eyes are fixed on the weight. Now here's the most important part: *Push your hips out to your right, and keep your right leg straight.* Bend from the hips and reach toward the floor with your left arm, while your chest turns to the right and your eyes stay on the weight. Touch the floor with your left hand, just inside your left foot. Here, in the finishing position, your arms and shoulders will form a straight line that's perpendicular to the floor. Reverse the steps as you return to the upright position. Do 5 to 8 reps with each arm overhead.

NOT READY FOR THIS ONE? Do the exercise as described with the weight in your left hand. You can use a much heavier weight, but don't treat this as a strength exercise. Work on your coordination and range of motion, with the goal of holding a weight overhead.

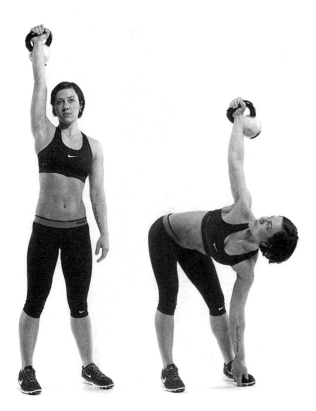

✳ Cable High to Low Chop

WHERE IT IS: Phase Three, Stage 9, Workout C

WHAT IT DOES: This progression from the previous chops employs a longer range of motion, and comes a little closer to mimicking the act of chopping wood, from which all these chops and lifts originate.

THE SETUP: Attach a D-shaped handle to the high cable pulley.

HOW TO DO IT: Grab the handle with both hands and stand sideways to the machine, with your feet shoulder-width apart and the handle just to the outside of the shoulder closest to the machine. Pull the handle down and across your torso so it ends up just past the hip farthest from the machine. Return to the starting position. Do 10 reps, switch sides, and repeat.

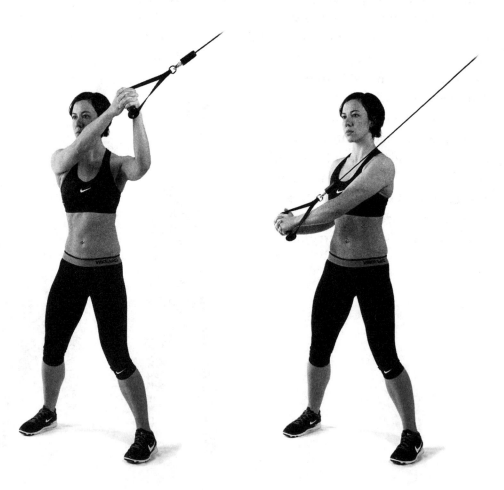

Lower-Body
Exercises

IN THE PREVIOUS CHAPTER, WE SHOWED you the core-training exercises in the order in which you do them in the program, starting with Stage 1, Workout A. But in this chapter, the exercises are shown by movement pattern and arranged from the most basic to the most advanced. The further you go in the program, the more leeway you have to choose your own exercise variations within each movement category.

The categories we use are admittedly arbitrary:

Squat: These are exercises in which your feet are parallel to each other, as they would be for a standing jump, and the weight is held somewhere above your waist, usually on your shoulders.

Deadlift: Alwyn refers to these exercises as *bend* or *hinge* movements. Others classify them as hip-dominant exercises, distinct from knee-dominant squats. It seems simplest to call them deadlifts, since every lifter immediately understands what you mean: your feet are parallel to each other, and you're lifting a weight that starts on the floor.

Other Hip Extension: Like the deadlift, the kettlebell swing is a *hip-extension* exercise, which means you straighten your body when it's bent forward at the hips. But although the muscle action is the same, the trajectory of the load is different—out and back vs. up and down. The other hard-to-classify exercise is the supine hip extension with leg curl, an occasional guest of the NROL series.

Squat-Deadlift Hybrids: If, for any reason, you can't do barbell squats or conventional deadlifts, Alwyn offers these alternatives, which you can substitute in either category.

Split Stance: These lunge-type exercises primarily work the quadriceps, but in different ways from the squats. With your feet separated, you have new balance and muscle-activation challenges.

Single Leg: More balance and activation challenges, but with all the force generated by one leg, instead of distributed to both. The exercises in this category work the posterior chain—the hamstrings, glutes, and back extensors.

SQUAT

All the squat variations should work the same muscles in about the same way. Your quadriceps and glutes are the prime movers, while your spinal erectors—the lower-back muscles that run alongside your spine—work extremely hard to stabilize your back. But it's best to think about the squat as a total-body exercise, one in which all your muscles work together to move the weight or provide stability.

✳ Goblet Squat

WHERE IT IS: Phase One, Stage 1, Workout A

WHAT IT DOES: It's the perfect introduction to the movement pattern. If it works for you, and you're getting stronger from workout to workout and stage to stage, you can use it throughout this program, in every phase. We encourage even the most experienced lifters to use it in Stage 1 and the Special Workout. If you've been doing heavy barbell squats, you can probably use a break.

THE SETUP: You can use a dumbbell, kettlebell, weight plate, or sandbag. Anything you can hold under your chin with both hands can work, as long as it allows you to increase the weight from week to week. If you're lifting something relatively heavy, you want to set it on a bench or box to begin. With a dumbbell, for example, you can set it upright on the end of a bench so you don't have to bend over so far to start each set.

HOW TO DO IT: Grab the weight with both hands and stand holding it under your chin and against your chest. Set your feet shoulder-width apart, with your toes pointed forward or angled out slightly. *Push your hips straight back*, as if aiming for a chair, and lower yourself until your thighs are parallel to the floor, or your elbows reach your knees. Rise back to the starting position and repeat.

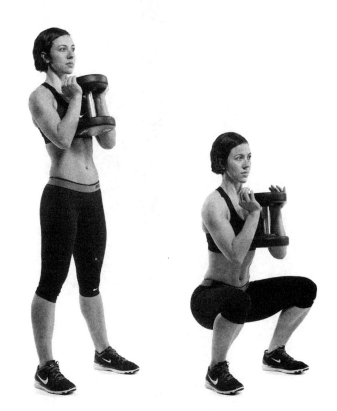

PRO TIP: "Spread the floor" with your feet. Of course you can't actually move the floor. The goal is to try to rotate your feet outward. This activates muscles on your outer hips, which in turn provide more stability to your core and even your knees.

GOBLET-SQUAT ALTERNATIVE

My favorite variation is the *kettlebell front squat*, an intermediate exercise between goblet squats with a dumbbell and front squats with a barbell. Grab a pair of kettlebells and lift them to your shoulders, holding them in the rack position, with your hands under your chin and the weights resting on the outside of your arms. From there, it's exactly like the front squat described next.

The challenge, as Alwyn points out, is that you need pairs of kettlebells that allow you to make steady progress. I'm lucky enough to train in a gym that has paired kettlebells in 2-kg increments up to 20 kg, which is 88 pounds for the pair. After that, they jump by 4 kg, which is almost 18 pounds per pair. A barbell allows you to add weight in smaller amounts.

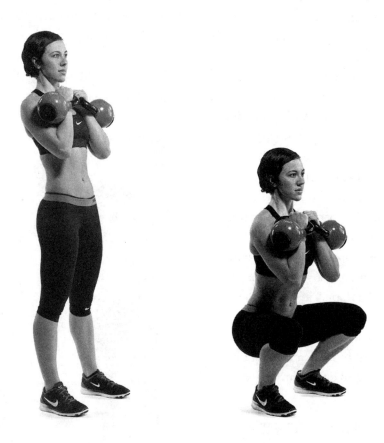

✳ Front Squat

WHERE IT IS: Phase One, Stage 2, Workout B

WHAT IT DOES: The front squat is the first progression from the goblet. It allows you to use heavier weights and to get used to a barbell on your shoulders.

THE SETUP: Set a barbell in a squat rack just below shoulder height.

HOW TO DO IT: Grab the bar with your hands about shoulder-width apart. Rotate your arms below and around the bar until your elbows point forward, your upper arms are parallel to the floor, and the bar rests on the front of your shoulders. Lift it off the supports and step back. Set your feet shoulder-width apart, with your toes pointed forward or angled out slightly. Push your hips back and lower your body until the tops of your thighs are parallel to the floor. Return to the starting position and repeat.

PICTURE THIS: Don't think about what your body looks like; instead, focus your eyes on a spot straight in front of you. Looking up or down could compromise your form.

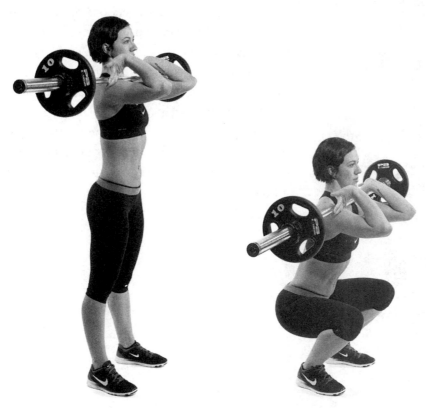

FRONT-SQUAT ALTERNATIVES

Front squats aren't for everybody. You can say that about any exercise, but the front squat can be especially vexing to some. In the photos we show the model holding the bar with a *clean grip*. It's the landing position of the bar in the clean, which

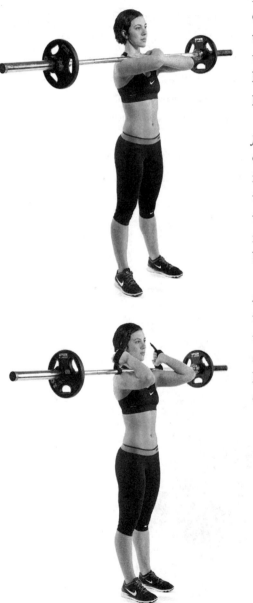

is the midpoint of the clean and jerk, one of the two Olympic lifts. To use a clean grip, you need to be able to roll the bar to the ends of your fingers while your upper arms remain parallel to the floor. Small hands, limited wrist flexibility, or any number of shoulder problems could make that a struggle.

The most popular alternative is the *cross-arm front squat*. You start with the same setup, but instead of grabbing the bar, you make a shelf for it by crossing your arms in front of your chest. The bar sits in the same place, between your front deltoids and your throat, only with your fingers on top instead of beneath it. It's a less stable position, but it's been used by bodybuilders going back to the 1960s, at least.

The better alternative is the *front squat with wrist straps*. (You can get a pair online for under $10.) Secure the straps to the bar, about shoulder-width apart, and then wrap them around your hands. Lift your elbows so your arms are parallel to the floor and perpendicular to your torso. Pull on the straps as you lift the bar off the rack.

✳ Back Squat

WHERE IT IS: Phase One, Stage 3, Workout B (with pause); Phase Two, Stage 4, Workout A (traditional)

WHAT IT DOES: Before you advance to using heavier weights, you want to make sure you can control the weight, rather than having the weight control you. The pause, used in Phase One, Stage 3, is especially important if this is your first time with a barbell on your back.

THE SETUP: Set a barbell in a squat rack just below shoulder height.

HOW TO DO IT: Grab the bar with your hands just outside shoulder width. Duck under the bar and squeeze your shoulder blades together. This flexes your upper traps, which gives the bar a platform to rest on. Lift the bar off the supports and step back. Set your feet about shoulder-width apart, with your toes pointed forward or angled out slightly. Push your hips back and descend as far as you can. If the workout calls for a pause, stop for 2 to 3 seconds in the bottom. Push back up to the starting position.

Don't allow your heels to rise off the floor. You need to keep your weight back.

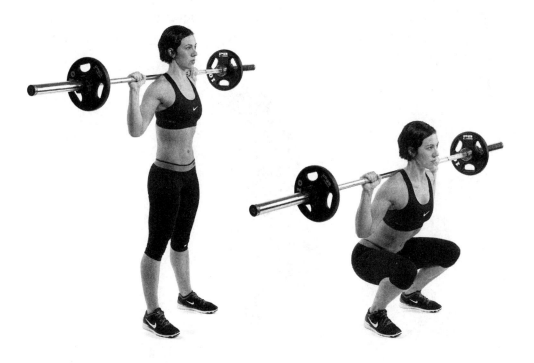

Safety Issues

Alwyn's view of the back squat is one of the biggest differences between *NROL for Women* and *Strong*. It allows you to lift heavier weights than any other squat variation, and if all else is equal, the heavier weight should do more to increase muscle mass and total-body strength. But problems arise when all else *isn't* equal. Here are some potential problems:

- Your upper arms are in the "double jeopardy" position: abducted (lifted up and away from your torso) and externally rotated (rolled back). If your shoulder mobility is limited or compromised by injury, the back squat can be brutal.
- With heavier weights, there's more compression on the knees than there is with the front squat. If you have any history of knee injuries, especially to the meniscus, you may want to skip the back squat.
- Many lifters, trying to achieve a deeper squat, will either bend farther forward or employ a "butt wink." It happens when your pelvis rotates backward, flattening the curve of your lumbar spine. Both modifications put you at greater risk for back injury.

Which brings us back to what we said earlier: *You don't have to do barbell squats to get all the benefits of Alwyn's program.* The goblet squat is the best variation for inexperienced lifters, and a great exercise for anyone, as long as your performance improves from week to week.

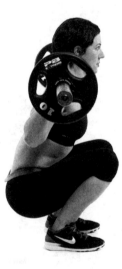

✳ Back Squat to Box with Pause

WHERE IT IS: Phase Two, Stage 6, Workout B

WHAT IT DOES: In a gym, you rarely see anyone squat with a heavy weight to the depth required in powerlifting competition, where the crease of the hip joint must be lower than the knee. So competitive lifters use the box squat to practice reaching legal depth. By pausing on the box you also break your momentum, which means you have to exert more effort to return to the starting position. Because it's harder, you can use less weight, which, as Alwyn says, actually makes it safer. Finally, the box helps you learn to sit back on a squat, which leads to a more upright posture.

THE BOX: If you want to practice competition depth, you'll need a box that's 10 to 12 inches high. (I'm 5 foot 10, and I need a 12-inch box.) But few lifters can achieve that depth immediately. So you'll need some way to start higher and then make adjustments as you improve. The best option is an adjustable box, which very few gyms will have. (You can buy one at elitefts.com for $200.) At powerlifting gyms, they often use mats or weight plates to adjust the height. That way different lifters can use the same box.

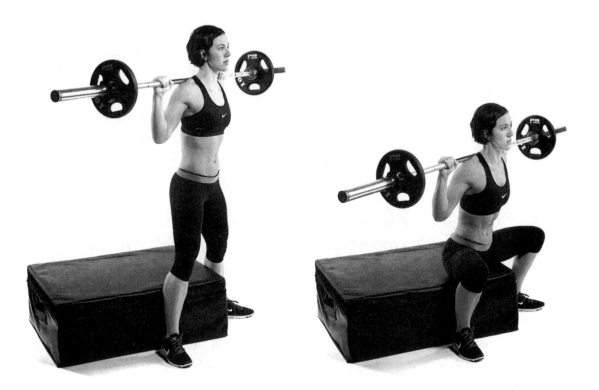

Safety Issues

- *Do not relax any muscles*, especially those in your lower back. Even with your butt on a sturdy box, you have to stay tight through your core and upper torso, as you would in any other squat.
- *Don't rock back on the box.* Powerlifters sometimes do this to generate momentum. It's sloppy and risky to your back.
- *Be cautious with your knees.* A 2012 study in the *Journal of Strength and Conditioning Research* found that the pressure on the knees is much higher in the box squat, compared to the traditional and powerlifting squats. (A traditional squat is the one shown in *Strong*. In the powerlifting squat, the bar sits lower on the back, and the torso tends to lean farther forward.)

THE SETUP: Position the box behind you in the squat rack and turn it so a corner points to the middle of your stance. Set the bar in the rack as you ordinarily would for a back squat.

BEFORE YOU LOAD THE BAR: Practice the movement with just your body weight at first. Then try it with an unloaded bar. Then do multiple warm-up sets before trying it with a training weight.

HOW TO DO IT: Lift the bar off the rack and step back so two sides of the box touch your calves. You'll probably take a wider-than-normal stance. *Sit back slowly* until you feel your glutes touch the box. Pause 2 to 3 seconds, and push back up to the starting position.

"Does It Have to Be a Barbell Back Squat? Can I Use Another Variation?"

Use whichever squat feels best for you. I did goblet box squats, and even with a lighter-than-normal weight it felt like a great exercise.

DEADLIFT

The act of lifting something heavy off the floor seems simple and intuitive only when you see it performed by someone who knows how to do it. In the hands of an unskilled lifter, a deadlift can be a strength coach's nightmare and a chiropractor's delight. I used to think the movement was self-correcting, that a poor lifter would get educated or get hurt before moving up to heavy weights. But just while writing these exercise chapters I saw two young guys in my gym lift serious loads with absolutely horrible form, bent in all the places that should be straight. That's why Alwyn now considers the barbell deadlift a more advanced movement, one that requires some time to learn.

✳ **Romanian Deadlift (RDL)**

WHERE IT IS: Phase One, Stage 2, Workout A

WHAT IT DOES: Novice lifters will get a chance to groove the hip-extension movement pattern without the challenge of pulling the weight from the floor. Those with more experience can use relatively heavy weights and focus on developing the glutes and hamstrings, which get more direct work in the RDL than in perhaps any other exercise in Alwyn's program.

THE SETUP: Set the barbell in a rack so it's a couple of feet above the floor.

HOW TO DO IT: Grab the bar with a shoulder-width, overhand grip. Lift it off the supports and step back, standing straight with the bar touching the front of your thighs. Set your feet so they're just inside your hands, with your toes pointed forward. *Push your hips back* and lower the bar until it's just below your knees, which will bend slightly. Now *thrust your hips forward* to return to the starting position.

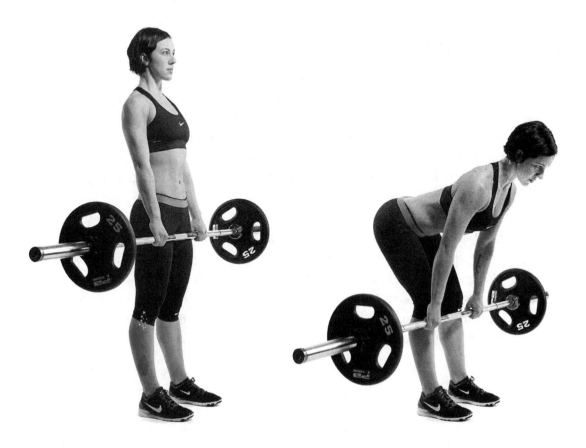

Why Your Chest Is the Key to a Good Deadlift

Chapter 12 explained how the lats work to stabilize your core. Now you get to put that knowledge into practice. How? By sticking your chest out. That forces your shoulders down, which activates your lats, which puts tension in the fascia of the lumbar region, which keeps your lower back and pelvis in the neutral position.

Someone standing in front of you should be able to see your chin, throat, and collarbones, at minimum. Some cleavage too, if your top allows it. If there's any writing on the shirt, that person should be able to read it, or at least see the tops of the letters.

A Quick Word About Your Neck

Sometimes you'll see a lifter hyperextend her neck on the deadlift. In response, coaches will cue that lifter to "tuck" her chin. But that would seem to contradict what I just wrote: that someone in front of you should be able to see your throat and collarbones. The best advice I've seen is to focus on a spot 10 to 15 feet in front of you, and keep your eyes focused on that spot throughout the lift. That puts your neck in the right position.

✳ Single-Arm Deadlift

WHERE IT IS: Phase One, Stage 3, Workout A

WHAT IT DOES: Lumbar stability is simple when the weight is evenly distributed. But when you're lifting with one arm instead of two, things change. The single-arm deadlift offers a coordination challenge to newer lifters, and an interesting, unusual way to improve total-body strength for veterans.

THE SETUP: Set a kettlebell on the floor. (A dumbbell variation is given in the options.)

HOW TO DO IT: Stand with your feet wide apart and the weight in between them. Bend at the hips and grab the handle with your nondominant hand (your left if you're right-handed). Push your hips back, tighten your core, and lift your chest. Now pull the weight straight up as you push your hips forward. Lower the weight to the floor, reset your body, and repeat. Do 8 reps, rest, and do the next exercise (dumbbell incline bench press). Rest, then do your second set of single-arm deadlifts, this time using your other arm. For the final set, do 4 reps with each arm.

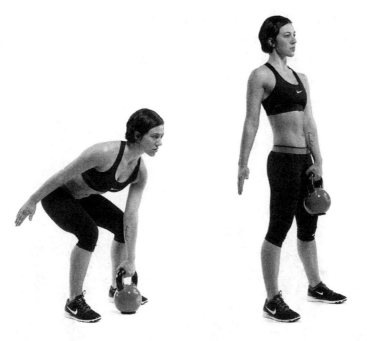

SINGLE-ARM OPTIONS

DUMBBELL: There are two ways to use a dumbbell. If you're new to lifting, start in the top position, push your hips back to lower the weight just past your knees, and then push your hips forward to finish the lift. More experienced lifters can start with the dumbbell on the floor. Position it in the middle of your stance, with the ends pointing toward your feet.

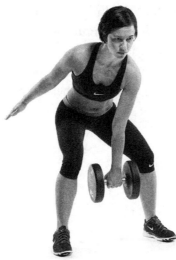

BARBELL: Here's a badass variation for stronger lifters: *barbell single-arm dead-lift.* You'll want to start with the bar at least 9 inches above the floor, as it would be with a 45-pound plate on each side. You can do that with bumper plates, as shown here, or by using smaller plates but starting with the bar elevated on blocks (as shown on the next page).

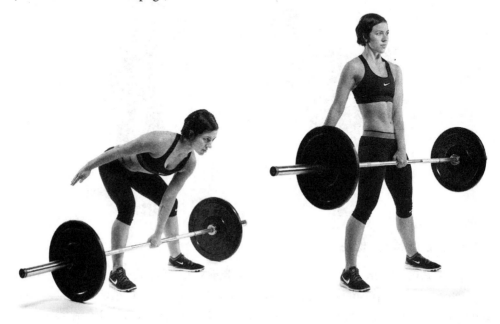

SUITCASE: You can do the *suitcase deadlift* with a dumbbell, kettlebell, or even a barbell. With a dumbbell, stand with the weight at your side. Push your hips back and squat down until the weight is just below your knee. Push your hips forward to return to the starting position. With a kettlebell or barbell, start with the weight on the floor, just outside your foot.

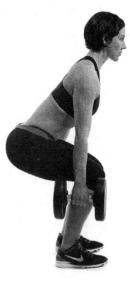

✳ Deadlift from Blocks

WHERE IT IS: Phase Two, Stage 4, Workout B

WHAT IT DOES: You'll practice true deadlifts—that is, lifting a weight from a dead stop—with a shorter range of motion.

THE SETUP: Set the barbell on blocks or supports so it's below your knees but at least mid-shin height.

HOW TO DO IT: Stand with your shins touching the bar, your feet shoulder-width apart, and your toes pointed forward or angled out slightly. Bend over and grab the bar with your hands just outside your legs. Push your hips back and your chest out, and tighten everything, starting with your grip. Pull the bar straight up as you push your hips forward. Lower it by pushing your hips back. Let the bar come to a complete stop on the supports. Reset your body and tighten your grip for the next lift.

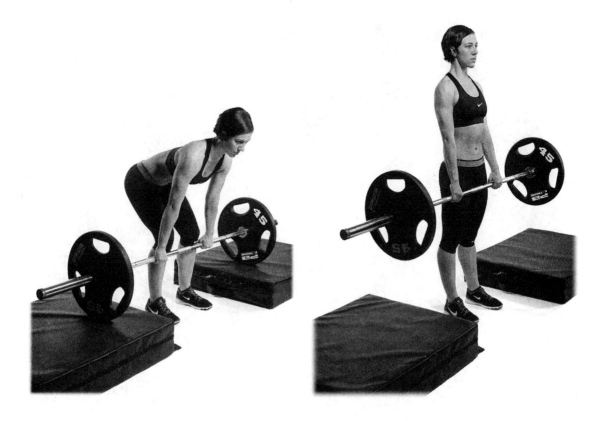

✳ Deadlift

WHERE IT IS: Phase Two, Stage 6, Workout B

WHAT IT DOES: Now that you've done all your prep work, you're ready to pull relatively heavy weights off the floor.

THE SETUP: Load a barbell and set it on the floor.

HOW TO DO IT: With your feet about shoulder-width apart and shins touching the bar, bend over and grab the bar with your hands just outside your legs. Hips back, chest out, everything tight. Pull the bar straight up as you push your hips forward. Lower it under control. Let the bar come to a complete stop before the next rep.

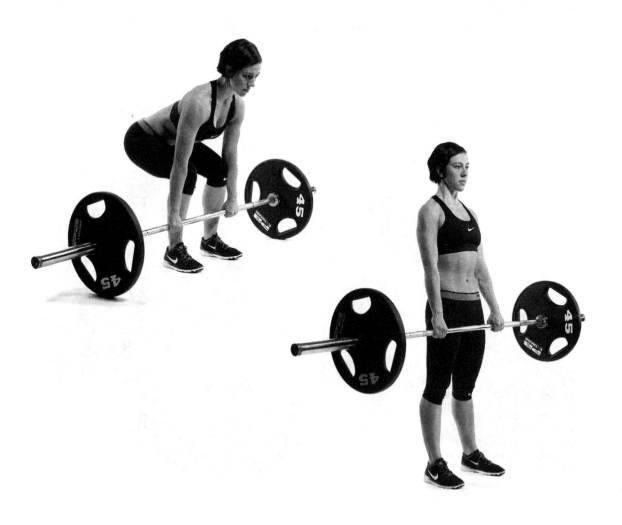

Grip Options

Alwyn recommends using the double-overhand grip on deadlifts for as long as you can. It allows your grip to get stronger along with everything else. But eventually, as you get into low-rep deadlifts with heavy weights, your grip will need some help. Our recommendations:

Chalk

You can find magnesium carbonite online and at select fitness-equipment stores. For those training at home or in a powerlifting gym, using it is never a problem. (One of the best things about training at home: You make your own rules. One of the worst things: You have to clean up your own mess.) Some gyms have rules against it, and I don't recommend breaking them. Not *flagrantly*, that is. If you're subtle, you can often get away with it. Carry a small amount in a travel soap dish, use only what you need for each set (no LeBron James clapping), and wipe everything down when you're finished.

Mixed Grip

Even with chalk, you'll hit your limits with the double-overhand grip. That's when you shift to a mixed grip: one hand over the bar and the other beneath. I recommend alternating hands, doing an equal number of reps with each hand over and under. I don't know how much difference it makes in muscle development, or joint stress, but it certainly feels different to me. If you're noticeably stronger with one combination, make sure you use it for your heaviest set.

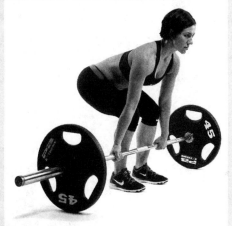

Straps

I mentioned lifting straps earlier, as a tool for front squats. They're most commonly used for deadlifts and barbell rows to get a few extra reps, and they're useful for advanced lifters, especially those with small hands. But do you *need* to get those extra reps? Here's Alwyn's take: "One of the most common complaints we hear is, 'My legs and back are fine, but my grip gives out.' I'm actually okay with your grip being the self-limiting factor in the deadlift. It's an excellent built-in safety mechanism."

OTHER HIP EXTENSION

✳ Kettlebell Swing

WHERE IT IS: Phase Two, Stage 5, Workout B

WHAT IT DOES: Most of us use the words *strength* and *power* interchangeably. But they mean different things. *Strength* can be measured simply: the most you can lift on any given exercise. The sport of powerlifting actually is a test of pure strength. *Power* is force times velocity, or the speed at which you can lift something. So Olympic weightlifting is a test of power as well as strength. The swing, although much simpler than an Olympic lift, is also a power exercise. The goal is to move the weight explosively, and for that explosive strength to translate to the deadlift, or any other hip-extension exercise.

WEIGHT SELECTION: If you've never done swings before, it's much more important to learn the exercise with a lighter weight vs. loading up and risking poor form. Standard advice is for women to start with 8 kg/18 pounds. (For men, it's 16 kg/35 pounds.)

THE SETUP: Put a kettlebell on the floor.

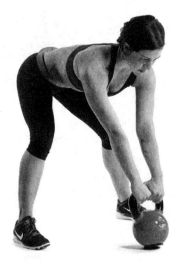

HOW TO DO IT: Stand over it with your feet a little beyond shoulder-width apart, your toes straight ahead or turned out slightly. Now take a step back. Bend forward at the hips and grab the handle with both hands, your thumbs touching, while keeping your back flat. (It should look like you're about to hike a football.) Pull the weight straight back between your legs. The entire kettlebell will end up behind you. Now thrust your hips forward, *throwing the bell out in front of you*. It should rise to chest level without any help from your shoulders. As soon as it stops rising, pull it back between your legs to begin the next swing.

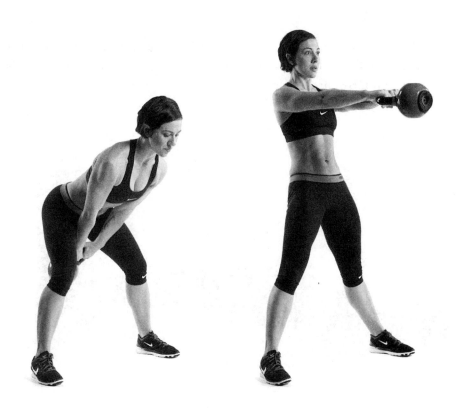

✳ Supine Hip Extension + Leg Curl (SHELC)

WHERE IT IS: Phase Three, Stage 7, Workout A

WHAT IT DOES: SHELC combines hip extension with *knee flexion*, better known as a leg curl. That second movement forces your hamstrings to do two jobs at once: straighten your hips and bend your knees. (You also work the largest calf muscle, the gastrocnemius, which assists with knee flexion.)

THE SETUP: You can do SHELC with a suspension system, Swiss ball, or Valslides. If you try it suspended, as shown here, set the handles to about knee height, and put your heels in the stirrups. With a Swiss ball, rest your heels on top of the ball. With Valslides, rest your heels on the discs. On all three, lie on your back on the floor, arms out to your sides.

HOW TO DO IT

SUSPENDED: Lift your hips so your body forms a straight line from torso to ankles. As you pull your heels toward your butt, raise your hips so your body forms a line from your torso through your knees.

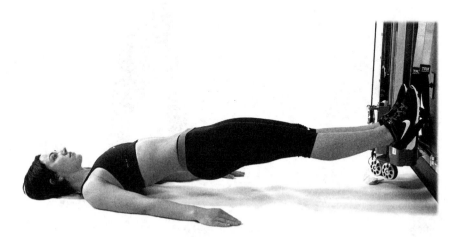

WITH VALSLIDES: Simultaneously lift your hips and bend your knees as you pull your heels toward your butt. At the top your body will form a straight line from torso to knees. Reverse the movement to return to the starting position.

WITH A SWISS BALL: Lift your hips until your body is straight from torso to ankles. Pull your heels toward your butt until you're straight from torso to knees. Straighten your legs and lower your hips until they almost touch the floor.

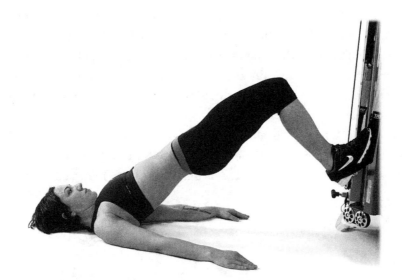

SQUAT-DEADLIFT HYBRIDS

You should never do an exercise that hurts. And barbell squats, to the front or back, hurt some of us. (Me, for example.) So where does that leave you? There's the goblet squat, of course. But as great an option as it is, some of you will be limited by the size of the dumbbells or kettlebells you have access to, as well as the amount of weight you can hold against your chest. The conventional deadlift is also difficult for some, especially if you have a history of lower-back problems.

If either or both of those movements is painful or forbidden by a doctor or therapist, Alwyn offers these two alternatives.

✳ Hex-Bar Deadlift

WHAT IT DOES: It gives you a way to lift a heavy weight off the floor without having to bend forward over the bar. Instead, the load is at the midline of your body. Because there's less bending forward, there's more bending of the knees. That puts it somewhere between a deadlift and a squat, only with less potential stress on your back and knees. Alwyn uses it as a squat substitute, but you can use it for either movement pattern.

THE BAR: A hex bar is a conventional barbell on the ends, where the weights go, but a six-sided hexagon on the middle. Most have high and low handles. The one shown in the photos is based on the original trap bar, a four-sided trapezoid, which

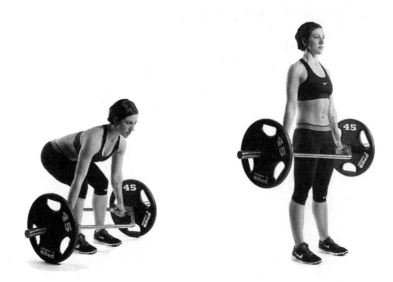

had only one set of handles. Weights vary, so if you're training at a gym, you'll need to ask someone how much it weighs.

THE SETUP: First decide if you want to use the low or high bars. Then load your weights. (If you change your mind, you can always flip the bar. Stand on one of the middle sections, grab the other middle section, and pull it toward you.) The low handles will be about 9 inches above the floor when you have a 45-pound plate on each side (or the equivalent, if you use bumper plates), which is the same as a deadlift. The high handles are 12 to 13 inches, making it more like a deadlift from blocks.

HOW TO DO IT: Stand in the middle, squat down, and grab the handles. Set your body as you would for a deadlift, with your back flat and chest up. Tighten everything. Now stand, pushing your hips forward to finish the lift. Push your hips back to lower the bar to the floor.

✳ Sumo Deadlift

WHAT IT DOES: Unlike the hex-bar deadlift, the sumo is an *actual* deadlift, one you can use in powerlifting competition. It allows you to pull from a wider stance, which reduces stress to your lower back and shifts some of the load to your quadriceps and adductors (inner-thigh muscles).

THE SETUP: Same as a conventional deadlift—just a bar on the floor.

HOW TO DO IT: Stand with your shins against the bar, taking an extremely wide stance, with your toes pointed out 45 degrees. Grab the bar in the middle, with your hands about shoulder-width apart. Push your hips back and chest up, and tighten everything, starting with your grip. Pull the weight straight up off the floor, keeping the bar as close to your body as you can. Push your hips back as you lower it.

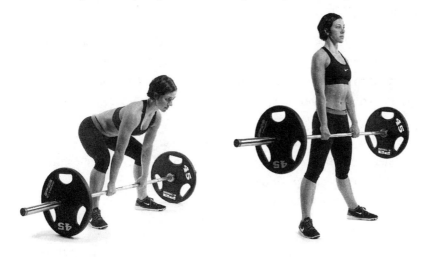

SPLIT STANCE

All the exercises in this category could be called split squats. Or, to use the official scientific term, *partial unilateral exercises.* And based on what we know about one of them (the one with the rear foot elevated on a bench), they work the same muscles as a barbell back squat, in more or less the same way, when done with similar intensity. This has been shown in at least two studies, one with young men and women who were novice lifters, and one with male football players and track and field athletes.

A Few Tips, Guidelines, and Reminders

- Your front leg is the "working" leg because it's doing almost all the work. The quadriceps are the prime movers, with minor assistance from the glutes and hamstrings.
- You probably want to start each set with your weaker leg forward (typically but not always your nondominant leg). Then do the same number of reps with your stronger leg. Whether you stop for rest in between depends on intensity and preference. For the hardest sets, you'll probably need to catch your breath.
- When both feet are on the floor—as in split squats and lunges—you want to keep your torso upright.
- When your back foot is off the floor—either suspended or resting on a bench—it's okay to lean forward. Each of us, depending on our leg bone lengths and proportions, will have slightly different form.

LOADING OPTIONS

Just about any type of resistance can work. Always start with just your body weight (which can be tougher than you expect on higher-rep sets), and then add what you need to keep it challenging. Confident lifters can get aggressive and push themselves hard. Your choices:

- Dumbbells or kettlebells held at arm's length at your sides
- Dumbbell, kettlebell, weight plate, or sandbag in the goblet position
- Kettlebells in the rack position
- A barbell in the front-squat position

- A barbell in the back-squat position
- Any of the aforementioned held overhead

✳ Split Squat

WHERE IT IS: Phase One, Stage 1, Workout B

WHAT IT DOES: This entry-level split squat gives you the most stable base because both feet remain on the floor and your body weight is evenly distributed.

HOW TO DO IT: If you're using just your body weight, stand with your hands in the prisoner grip (fingers touching behind your head). If you need to add resistance, you can use any of the choices I just listed under "Loading Options." With your feet hip-width apart, take a long step back with your right leg. From this starting position, lower your body until the top of your left thigh is parallel to the floor and your right knee nearly touches the floor. Rise back to the starting position. Do all your reps, switch legs, and repeat.

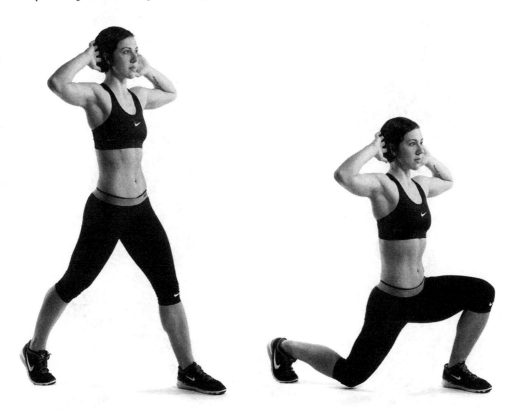

✳ Reverse Lunge

WHERE IT IS: Phase One, Stage 2, Workout A

WHAT IT DOES: The reverse lunge is one of the most versatile exercises you can do. If you've never lifted before, you'll quickly get the hang of it. An advanced lifter can put a heavy barbell on her shoulders and work her lower-body muscles as thoroughly as she would in a squat, while using less than half the load. No matter your experience or strength, your goal is the same: Do as much work as you can within the parameters of Alwyn's program.

HOW TO DO IT: Grab whatever form of resistance you choose (see "Loading Options" on p. 190) and stand with your feet hip-width apart. Take a long step back with one leg and lower yourself until the top of your front thigh is parallel to the floor and your rear knee nearly touches the floor. Step back to the starting position. Do all your reps, switch legs, and repeat.

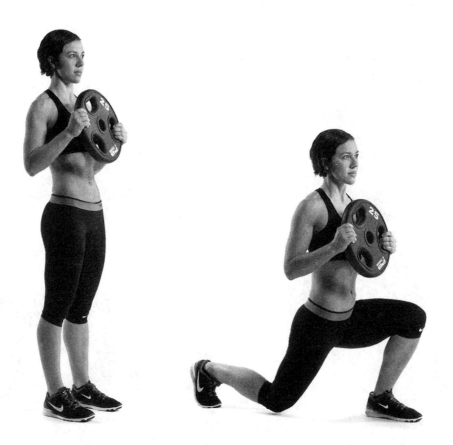

✳ Suspended Lunge and Touch

WHERE IT IS: Phase One, Stage 2, Workout B

WHAT IT DOES: Alwyn regards the suspended lunge with touch as a hybrid of the split-stance exercises in this section and the single-leg exercises shown next, with a lot of work for the glutes and less for the quadriceps.

THE SETUP: Combine the stirrups of a suspension system and lower the handles to mid-calf height.

HOW TO DO IT: Put your right foot in the stirrups and hop forward with your left foot until your right knee is bent about 90 degrees and your right shin is more or less parallel to the floor. Your thighs will be alongside each other, with your hips and shoulders square and facing forward. Bend your left knee and lower your body as far as you can while keeping your balance. Touch the floor with your right hand at the bottom. Rise back to the starting position. Do all your reps, switch sides, and repeat.

NO SUSPENSION SYSTEM? Do the single-leg Romanian deadlift (described on p. 201).

BADASS OPTION: At the top of each rep, do a hop with your working leg. So you descend, touch the floor, rise, hop, land, begin the next rep.

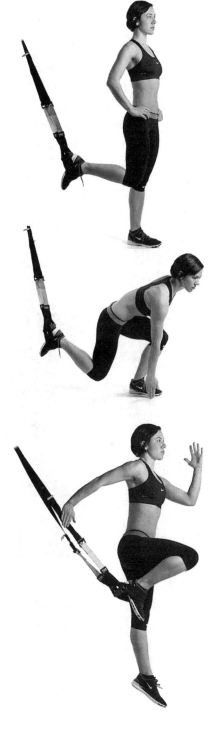

✳ Suspended Lunge

WHERE IT IS: Phase Two, Stage 6, Workout A

HOW TO DO IT: Same as the suspended lunge with touch, only you'll do a running motion with your arms—with your left leg forward, drive your right arm up as you descend, and your left arm forward as you rise. If you're comfortable with the motion, try holding light dumbbells.

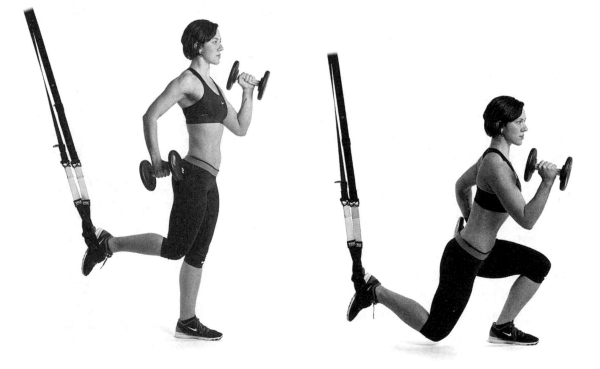

✳ Rear-Foot-Elevated Split Squat (RFESS)

WHERE IT IS: Phase One, Stage 3, Workout A

WHAT IT DOES: Now we're into serious badass territory, and yet the RFESS is versatile enough for anyone who's made it to Stage 3 without retreating to the circuit of machines on the other side of the gym. But it should never be easy. As Alwyn points out, your legs never really get a break, as they do at the top of a bilateral squat. Your working leg is always under some level of tension, and that extra stress on your muscles adds up.

THE SETUP

PART 1. THE BOX: You'll need a box, step, or bench to rest the foot of your nonworking leg. There's no rule for how high the step must be. You just want your working leg to end up parallel to the floor in the bottom position. If you've never done the exercise before, start with a low step, perhaps 6 to 8 inches high. You'll set your toes on it. More advanced readers can use a box or bench 12 to 18 inches high, on which you'll rest the instep of your nonworking foot.

PART 2. THE LOAD: Those doing RFESS for the first time should start with their body weight and use an external load only if they get all the reps with both legs on every set. Others need to choose something from the list on p. 190. Most readers will use dumbbells, as shown in the photos.

For advanced lifters who decide to use a barbell, set it up as you would for a back squat, with the box or bench behind you. With the bar on your shoulders, you'll step back, and then very carefully lift your nonworking leg and set the foot on the box.

HOW TO DO IT: Once you're set up as described, with the toes or instep of your rear leg on the box or bench, descend until the thigh of your working leg is parallel to the floor. Push back up. Do all your reps, switch legs, and repeat.

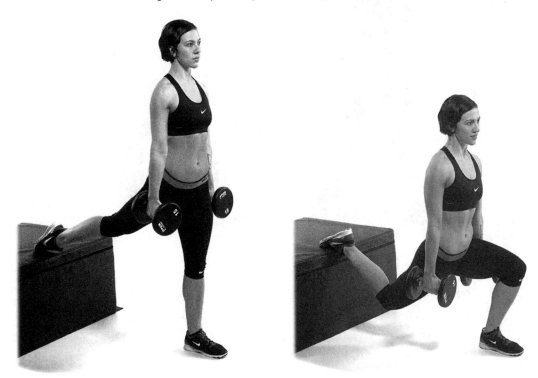

✳ Side Lunge and Touch

WHERE IT IS: Phase Two, Stage 4, Workout B

WHAT IT DOES: Lunge variations have a useful way of calling your attention to muscles you didn't know you have or reminding you of muscles you've neglected. The side lunge will probably do both. It targets your adductors, but the unbalanced load—a single weight in the hand opposite the working leg—brings countless stabilizing muscles into play.

HOW TO DO IT: Hold a dumbbell in your right hand at arm's length as you stand with your feet wide apart, toes pointed forward. Lean to your left, push your hips back, and drop into a deep squat as you touch the floor with the weight just inside your left foot. In the bottom position, your left thigh will be parallel to the floor, with your left shin close to perpendicular, your right leg straight, both feet flat on the floor, and your shoulders and hips facing forward.

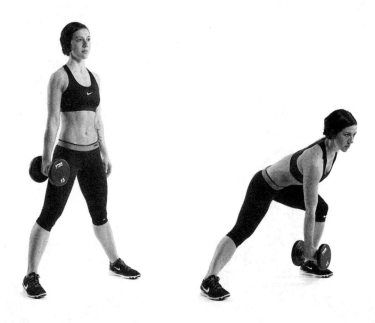

✳ Forward Lunge

WHERE IT BECOMES AN OPTION: Phase Three, Stage 7, Workout B

WHAT IT DOES: The forward lunge is what most of us would call a lunge, with no modifier. After all, if you're reading a news story, and you're told that a suspect "lunged" at a policeman, you don't picture him doing a split squat or stepping backward. The word has obvious connotations. But in a strength workout, the most obvious lunge variation isn't the one you want to start with. To Alwyn, it's an advanced exercise, testing not just your strength but also your balance and the integrity of your knee joints. Even the most skilled lifters might be better served with another option. That's why, whenever you see "lunge" in the Phase Three programs, you can use the forward lunge, reverse lunge, or anything else in the split-squat category.

HOW TO DO IT: Choose a loading option from the list on p. 190. Stand holding the weight with your feet hip-width apart. Take a long step forward and descend until your front leg is parallel to the floor and the knee of your trailing leg nearly reaches the floor. Push back to the starting position. You can do all your reps with one leg, then switch legs and repeat, or alternate until you've done all the reps with both legs.

SINGLE LEG

All the exercises in this category can be classified as hip-dominant. Single-leg deadlifts and hip thrusts are pure hip-extension exercises. Step-ups involve some movement at the knee and ankle joints, which bring more lower-body muscles into play. But the glutes still get more work than the quadriceps or hamstrings. You won't find as many exercise descriptions here as you did for the squat, deadlift, and split-stance categories. But that doesn't mean you lack options, especially on the step-up. With all the different ways to load it, you can always keep the exercise fresh.

✴ Step-Up

WHERE IT IS: Phase One, Stage 1, Workout A

WHAT IT DOES: The squat has a reputation as an exercise that hits all the lower-body muscles. But the step-up may actually be the superior all-around muscle builder, at least according to a study at Marquette University. The researchers used 15 female athletes (at least one of whom was a pro soccer player), and had them work with heavy weights and an 18-inch step. (The women averaged 5 feet, 5 inches tall.) They found that the subjects' glutes were much more active on step-ups compared to squats, and the hamstrings worked moderately harder.

THE SETUP: You need a box or step high enough to challenge you and solid enough to support you. If you have any history of knee or hip problems, I recommend a low step—8 to 12 inches.

HOW TO DO IT: With one or more weights in one or both hands, stand facing the step. Place your left foot on it, flat, with your right foot on the floor. *Press down through your left heel* to lift yourself up until your right leg is even with your left. Brush the step with your right foot, but don't use it to support any part of your weight. Lower your right foot back to the floor. Do all your reps with your left leg, then switch legs and repeat.

LOADING OPTIONS

As with the split-stance exercises, you have lots of choices:

- Dumbbells or kettlebells held at arm's length at your sides
- A single dumbbell or kettlebell held at arm's length on the same side as the working leg (the one stepping up)
- A single dumbbell held alongside your shoulder on the same side as the working leg
- Two kettlebells in the rack position or a single kettlebell held in the rack position on the same side as the working leg
- Two dumbbells or kettlebells held overhead
- A single dumbbell or kettlebell held overhead on the side opposite the working leg (your right hand when stepping up with your left leg)
- A barbell in the back-squat position
- A barbell, weight plate, or sandbag held overhead

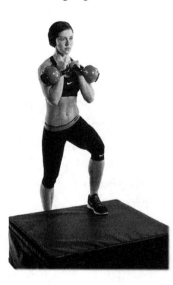
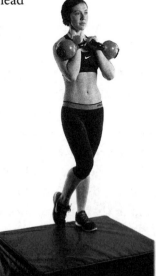

✴ Single-Leg Romanian Deadlift (RDL) with Reach

WHERE IT IS: Phase One, Stage 1, Workout B

WHAT IT DOES: The single-leg RDL develops strength in your glutes and hamstrings, stability in your back and hips, and, more obviously, balance while standing on one leg. This entry-level version teaches you the basic movement pattern before you try it with weights.

HOW TO DO IT: Stand with your feet hip-width apart. Lean forward at the hips while extending your right leg straight back behind you, reaching forward with your right arm, and supporting your weight on your left leg. As you reach the finishing position, your right arm and right leg will align with your torso, while your left leg is straight and perpendicular to the floor. Squeeze your left glute to pull you back to the starting position. Do all your reps, then switch sides and repeat, extending your left arm and leg and supporting your weight on your right leg.

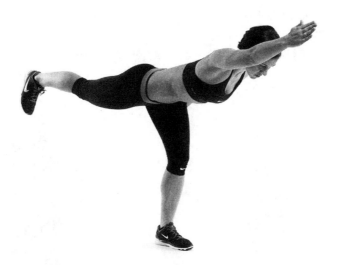

"Seriously? This Is an *Exercise*?"

Too easy? No problem. If you get all the reps on the first set, add weight for the next set, using either of the suggested variations.

✴ Single-Leg Romanian Deadlift from Box

WHERE IT IS: Phase One, Stage 3, Workout B

WHAT IT DOES: This intermediate step gets you accustomed to lifting a weight while shortening the range of motion. The goal is to ensure you do the movement well before you try it with a challenging load.

THE SETUP: You'll need a dumbbell or kettlebell and a box or step that's 8 to 12 inches high—higher for the dumbbell, lower for the kettlebell. Set the weight on the box.

HOW TO DO IT: Stand with the inside of your left foot alongside the box and the toes of your right foot directly behind it. Bend forward at the hips, extending your right leg behind you, as you reach down and grab the weight with your right hand. At this point your torso and right leg will be aligned and form a 45-degree angle with your left leg. Lift the weight off the box as you squeeze your left glute and pull yourself back to the starting position. Bend again at the hips as you lower the weight toward the box. Stop just short of touching it. Continue until you finish all your reps. After the final rep, set the weight on the box, switch positions, and repeat with the weight in your left hand and your right leg doing the work.

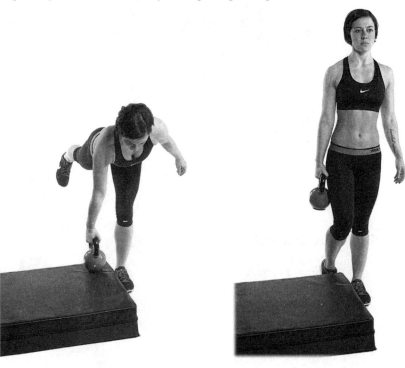

✳ Single-Leg Romanian Deadlift

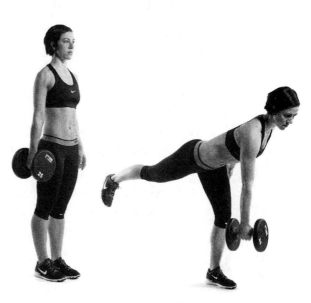

WHERE IT IS: Phase Two, Stage 5, Workout A

WHAT IT DOES: The single-leg RDL allows you to use relatively heavy weights through the full range of motion. Although the focus is on the glutes and hamstrings, don't discount the benefit of strengthening the smaller muscles in your torso and legs, especially the ones that provide stability to your ankle joints.

HOW TO DO IT: Stand holding a dumbbell or kettlebell in your right hand. Bend forward at the hips as you extend your right leg behind you, with your right arm straight as you lower the weight toward the floor. Bend as far as your balance will allow. Squeeze your left glute and return to the starting position. Do all your reps, switch sides, and repeat.

PICTURE THIS: You don't have to go as far as we show in the photos, with your torso and right leg parallel to the floor; the key is to keep your neck, torso, and right leg in a straight line, with your shoulders and hips square to the floor.

BADASS OPTION: For lower-rep sets, try it with a barbell, holding it with both hands. It's a very different challenge to your balance and stability.

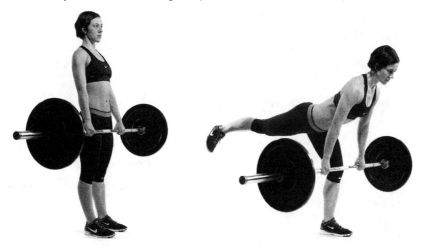

✳ Single-Leg Hip Thrust

WHERE IT IS: Phase Three, Stage 8, Workout A

WHAT IT DOES: It's an optional exercise designated for Stage 8, but one you can use at other points in the program if you get tired of the other single-leg choices. Or you can skip it and continue using step-ups and single-leg RDLs. The hip thrust more directly targets your glutes, without as many moving parts as the step-up or the balance component of the RDL.

THE SETUP: You just need a bench and a little space to the side of it.

HOW TO DO IT: Sit with your body perpendicular to the bench and the middle of your back resting against one side. Set your left foot on the floor and lift your right leg. Squeeze your left glute and raise your hips until your body is straight from your neck to your left knee, your left shin is perpendicular to the floor, and your right leg is more or less aligned with your torso. Lower your hips, do all your reps, then switch legs and repeat.

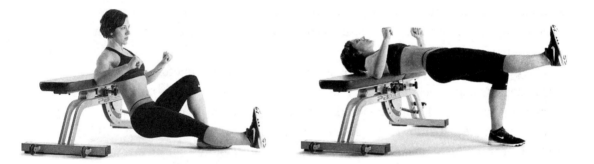

LOADING OPTIONS

Once you have the hang of the movement, you can add weight a bunch of ways:

- A dumbbell, sandbag, heavy chains, weighted vest, or even a small child on your lap
- A resistance band across your lap, with the loops attached to something sturdy on either side of you (some heavy-duty squat racks have cleats for band exercises)
- A barbell across your lap; if you choose this super-badass option, make sure you have a thick pad between the bar and your pelvis

Upper-Body Exercises

Unlike the lower-body exercises in Chapter 13, upper-body exercises fall into just two categories: pushes (push-ups and chest and shoulder presses) and pulls (rows, chin-ups, and pulldowns). Pushes primarily work the chest, shoulders, and triceps. Pulls hit the lats, trapezius, rear shoulders, and biceps. But all of them, done correctly, turn into total-body lifts. Your core provides stability, and your hips and legs provide the platform that makes heavy upper-body lifts safe and productive.

PUSH

Pushing exercises are usually classified as horizontal (push-ups and bench presses) or vertical (overhead presses and inverted push-ups). Or you can call the former "chest presses" and the latter "shoulder presses," and everyone will know exactly what you mean. The idea is that these are two clearly delineated movement patterns, with different muscle groups acting as the prime movers. What I find interesting is how little difference there is, at least in my own experience.

Back in 2005, as Alwyn and I put the finishing touches on the original *NROL*, I did the last serious strength program my middle-aged body allowed. I'd hoped to set a new personal record in the barbell bench press, but had failed to even match my previous record, set three years earlier. A few days later I went into the gym to do a lighter workout, using dumbbells. But the lighter weights felt *too* light. I worked my way up the rack until I had a new personal record in the dumbbell bench press, despite the fact I hadn't done any dumbbell presses for months. Before the workout was over I set another personal record, this time in the dumbbell shoulder press. I hadn't done any overhead presses at all during the three-month strength program.

I've noticed the same phenomenon with other exercises that we tend to think of as unrelated. If I build strength in rowing exercises, it translates to chin-ups, and strength in chin-ups crosses over to rows. Powerlifters will tell you that building strength in the squat improves your performance in the deadlift.

Strength is strength. Where we see separations, our bodies see a continuum. We believe in specificity—we must do *this* to achieve *this*—but human physiology prefers overlap.

Alwyn still gives you lots of options, with different angles and grips. It's not so much to develop strength at those specific angles or to preferentially work certain muscle fibers. The goal is to keep your workouts fresh and to minimize the risk of overuse injuries in your shoulder joints.

✳ Push-Up

WHERE IT IS: Phase One, Stage 1, Workout A

WHAT IT DOES: It's the alpha press: the first and best choice to develop strength in your chest, shoulders, and triceps, while simultaneously improving core stability and even some strength in your serratus, the muscles that pull your shoulder blades apart.

HOW TO DO IT (CLASSIC PUSH-UP): Get into push-up position (startling, right?), with your weight balanced on your hands and toes. Your hands are directly beneath your shoulders, your feet are hip-width apart, and your body forms a straight line from neck to ankles. Bend your elbows and *lower your body as a unit* until your chest is a couple of inches from the floor, your upper arms are even with your torso, or your chest touches carpet, whichever comes first. Push back up to the starting position.

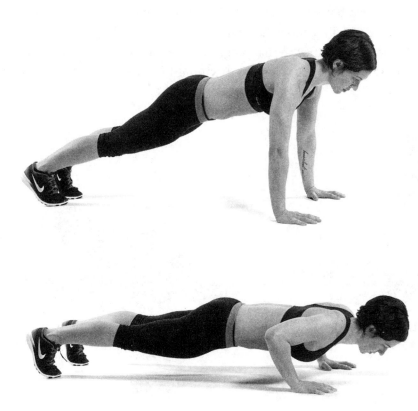

PUSH-UP OPTIONS AND VARIATIONS: When I asked the women in a Facebook group about push-ups, I got a bigger range of responses than I expected. At the high end were multiple women who can do 25 to 35 per set, and one who said she does 101 a night. (She didn't say how many sets it takes, just that she always hits that number.) Others said they still can't do one. All of them were actively training and were either doing or had completed at least one of Alwyn's NROL programs.

So I knew I had my work cut out for me. Let's start with a look at why the exercise is so challenging to many women:

In the classic push-up, you're lifting the equivalent of two-thirds of your body weight. Even in the "girl" push-up, with your knees on the floor, you're lifting about 50 percent. Thus for a 140-pound woman, a classic push-up is similar to a 90-pound bench press. Even guys, with their biological advantage in upper-body strength, struggle to reach double-digit push-up reps with good form.

NOT READY FOR THIS ONE? Do the *push-up with hands elevated* on a box or bench. On a 24-inch box, you're lifting the equivalent of 40 percent of your weight. On a 12-inch box, it's a little more than half. Start with as much elevation as you need to complete the reps specified in that program—even if it means you're just leaning forward against a wall. Work your way down until you can do push-ups from the floor.

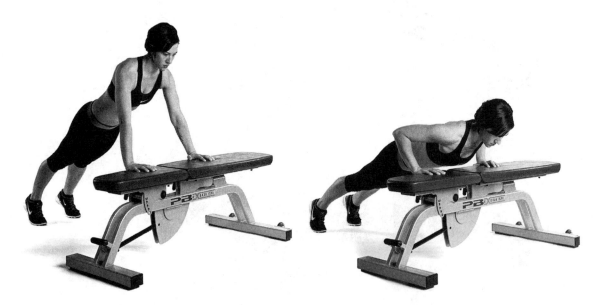

BADASS OPTION: Do *push-ups with feet elevated*. With your feet on a 12-inch box, the load has been estimated to be 70 percent of your weight. At 24 inches, it's about 75 percent. The muscles that stabilize your shoulder blades, including your trapezius and serratus, get more work as well.

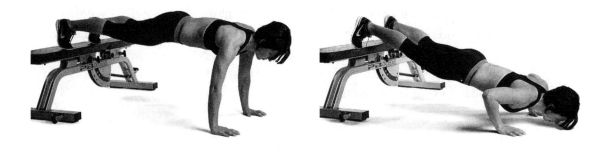

Depending on the equipment you have available, you can also do *push-ups with a weighted vest*, or even with chains. Some readers have told me they have a training partner put weight plates on their back, which seems both uncomfortable and dangerous to me. But if it works for *you* . . .

IF YOU NEED VARIETY: Stage 1 calls for push-ups in workouts A and B. To give yourself some variety, in the B workout you can use the *pike push-up*: Lift your hips as high as you can, then lower your shoulders toward the floor. It's the body-weight equivalent of an incline bench press.

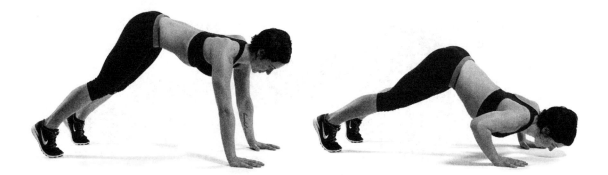

For a badass variation on the pike, elevate your feet. For a badass-squared option, try the *inverted push-up*: With your toes on a stack of boxes, set yourself up so your torso is perpendicular to the floor. It's kinda-sorta like doing a shoulder press, only with a lot of blood rushing to your forehead.

You can also shift the emphasis to your triceps with the *narrow-base push-up*. Set up for a classic push-up, only with your hands inside shoulder width. I wouldn't recommend it if you have any history of elbow injuries because there's more strain on those joints. Interestingly, a couple of studies have shown that the pectoral muscles are also more active with your hands closer together. Conversely, the farther apart you set your hands, the less elbow strain you'll incur, but the less work you'll give to both your chest and triceps.

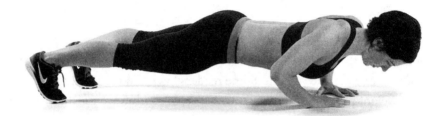

Finally, you can elevate your feet on an unstable surface: *Push-ups with feet suspended* are a great choice, as are *push-ups with feet on a Swiss ball*. Although there's no difference in chest or triceps muscle activation compared to elevating your feet on a stable surface, core-muscle activation should increase.

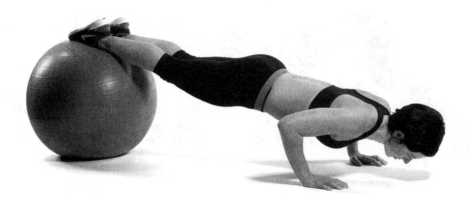

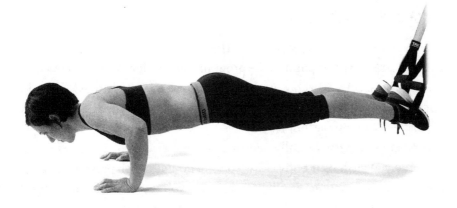

"What If My Boobs Get in the Way?"

I never would've thought of this one, but a couple of readers have told me that women with large breasts can't always do classic push-ups. There's a hard stop that might be several inches short of the full range of motion. The solution is *push-ups with your hands on boxes*—one on each side, with extra room for your breasts in between. Don't do this to extend the normal range of motion. You just want your upper arms to be parallel to the floor in the bottom position. Any deeper and you potentially put your shoulder joints at risk.

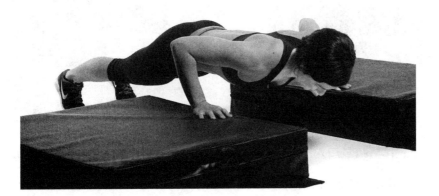

✳ Dumbbell Bench Press

WHERE IT IS: Phase One, Stage 2, Workout B

WHAT IT DOES: By this point in the program, you've done push-ups in both Stage 1 workouts, the Special Workout, and Stage 2, Workout A. My guess? You're kind of tired of push-ups. (I'm intuitive that way.) So now you get to do the equivalent with dumbbells. It seems simple, but it's not.

The push-up is what we call a *closed-chain exercise*. Your hands are in a fixed position, and you push your body away from them. The bench press is an *open-chain exercise*. The muscle actions are the same, but if you watch a teen or senior do the exercise for the first time, you'll appreciate how difficult it can be to control two objects that seem to have their own agenda.

THE SETUP: You just need a flat bench and a pair of dumbbells.

HOW TO DO IT: Grab the weights and lie on your back on the bench with your feet on the floor and at least shoulder-width apart. Start with the weights straight up over your shoulders, palms out. You want your head, shoulders, and glutes touching the bench, with an arch in your lower back. Lower the weights toward the edges of your shoulders, then press them back up to the starting position.

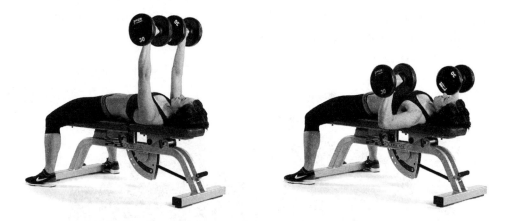

"What If My Feet Don't Touch the Floor? Can I Put Them on the Bench?"

Alwyn doesn't like that adjustment, for two reasons: First, it flattens your lower back, which is an unnatural position for lifting. Second, it takes away the balance your legs provide. You end up with more pressure on your shoulder joints and less support from your core and lower body. It's better to use the incline bench press, shown next, with your feet on the floor.

✳ Dumbbell Incline Bench Press

WHERE IT IS: Phase One, Stage 3, Workout A

WHAT IT DOES: By raising the bench, you shift the emphasis to the upper fibers of your pectorals and give more work to your deltoids. For some lifters this angled press feels better for the shoulder joints.

THE SETUP: Set a bench to an incline between 30 and 45 degrees.

HOW TO DO IT: Grab the weights and lie on your back on the bench with your feet flat on the floor. Start with the weights straight up over your shoulders, palms out, with your head, shoulders, and butt in contact with the bench. Lower the weights to your shoulders, then press back to the starting position.

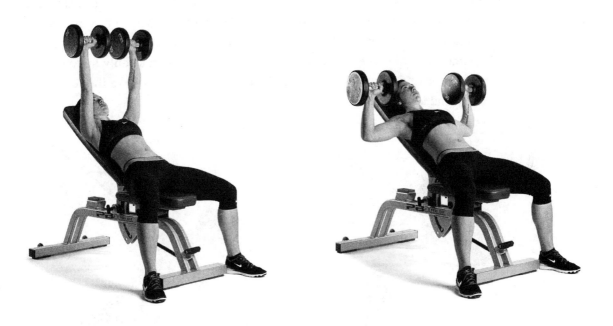

✳ Suspended Push-Up

WHERE IT IS: Phase One, Stage 3, Workout B

WHAT IT DOES: Remember a few pages ago when I described all the push-ups you've done so far? For a reward, you get to do . . . another kind of push-up! But it's one with quite a bit more core-muscle activation.

THE SETUP: Set the handles of a suspension system somewhere between knee and mid-thigh height. (The higher they are, the easier it will be.)

HOW TO DO IT: Grab the handles and lean forward, with your body straight from neck to ankles and your weight supported by your toes and the straps of the suspension system. Your arms are out in front of you at a 90-degree angle to your torso. Bend your elbows and lower your body as a unit until your upper arms are parallel to the floor. Push back up to the starting position.

DON'T HAVE A SUSPENSION SYSTEM? You can put your hands on any unstable surface. This is probably the only appropriate use of a BOSU ball in one of Alwyn's programs. (Put your hands on the platform, rather than the ball.) In the past we've recommended doing push-ups with your hands on a Swiss ball, but in my experience that's a little *too* unstable. Your core gets a lot of work at the expense of your prime movers—your chest, shoulders, and triceps. If that's your only option, I recommend pushing the ball against a wall. To me, it seems more like the suspended push-up and less like a circus trick.

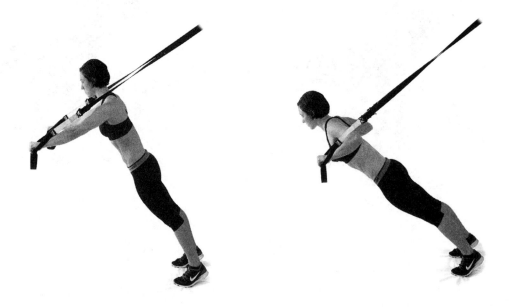

✳ Dumbbell Single-Arm Push Press

WHERE IT IS: Phase Two, Stage 5, Workout B

WHAT IT DOES: All the pushing exercises so far have been with two arms. Now, with the first overhead press in Alwyn's program, you get the challenge of using one arm in a total-body lift. Like the kettlebell swing in Chapter 13, it's a combination strength-and-power exercise, with a core challenge added in.

THE SETUP: You just need a single dumbbell (or, if you're feeling adventurous, a kettlebell).

HOW TO DO IT: Stand with the dumbbell in one hand at shoulder level, your palm turned in. Drop your knees a few inches, as if you were going to jump, and as you come up, push the weight overhead. Immediately drop back down for the next rep. Do all your reps, then switch sides and repeat.

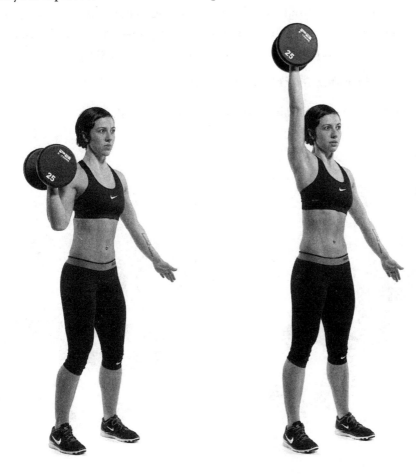

✳ Barbell Incline Bench Press

WHERE IT IS: Phase Two, Stage 6, Workout A

WHAT IT DOES: If you've never done a barbell bench press, this variation will help you decide if it's right for you. Otherwise, it works the chest, shoulders, and triceps the same way as the dumbbell version.

THE SETUP: Back in the day, every gym with free weights also had an incline barbell bench press station. If your current gym doesn't, or if you train at home, you'll have to set your bench up inside a power rack. I recommend starting with a 45-degree incline, and then adjusting the supports so the bar sits just below arm's length when you're positioned for the lift.

HOW TO DO IT: Lie on your back on the bench, with your head, shoulders, and glutes touching it and your feet flat on the floor. Grab the bar with an overhand, shoulder-width grip and your thumbs wrapped around it. Lift it off the supports (or have a spotter hand it to you), and tighten everything up—grip, shoulders, core, legs. Lower the bar to the top of your chest, and push back to the starting position.

"What If This One Doesn't Work for Me?"

No problem. Do the dumbbell incline bench press instead.

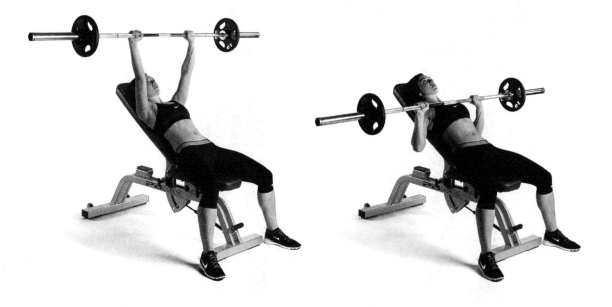

✳ Dumbbell Neutral-Grip Bench Press

WHERE IT IS: Phase Two, Stage 6, Workout B

WHAT IT DOES: The neutral grip—palms facing each other—will bring your elbows in closer to your torso. It's a more stable position, which means you'll *probably* be able to work with heavier weights, and *possibly* see more overall chest development, with perhaps a little less work for your shoulders and triceps (which will get plenty of work on the incline bench press).

THE SETUP: Just dumbbells and a flat bench.

HOW TO DO IT: Lie on your back on the bench, holding the weights straight up over your chest with your palms turned in. Lower the weights to the sides of your chest and then push back to the starting position.

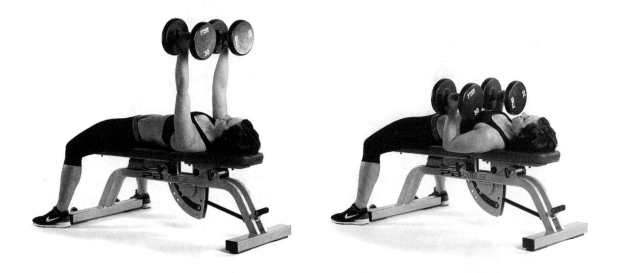

PHASE THREE PRESS OPTIONS AND VARIATIONS

In Stages 7, 8, and 9, Workout B, Alwyn has you do a press for low reps, with heavy weights. But he doesn't specify which press. Your options include:

- Dumbbell flat or incline bench press
- Barbell flat or incline bench press
- Dumbbell shoulder press
- Barbell shoulder press

You can use the same one for all three stages or switch them up. In my experience, as I suggested earlier, strength in barbell lifts should translate to dumbbells. But it probably won't go the other direction. Barbell lifts are technically more complex, and they also depend more on individual biomechanics. Someone with shorter arms and a thicker torso will be much better at the barbell bench press than a leaner, longer-limbed lifter. (The longer-armed person has an advantage in the deadlift because her range of motion will be shorter.)

But the most important factor is safety. If an exercise is uncomfortable now, it'll only get worse. That's especially true for the barbell bench press. There's no question it builds muscle and increases upper-body strength. There's also no question that a lot of lifters develop chronic shoulder problems. As Alwyn once told me, "The flat barbell bench press pretty much wrecks every shoulder joint eventually."

The open question is whether the rewards are bigger than the risks *for you*. Not for me or Alwyn or your powerlifting friends or anyone else. You're not a statistic. You're a physiologically unique person who might have healthy shoulders and an ideal frame for this exercise. Or you might not. Whatever you choose, remember that there's always an alternative to an exercise that doesn't fit your body.

✳ Barbell Bench Press

THE SETUP: If you have a bench with uprights, you're good to go. If not, you'll need to set the supports of a rack to the right height for you.

HOW TO DO IT: Grab the bar overhand, your thumbs wrapped around the bar

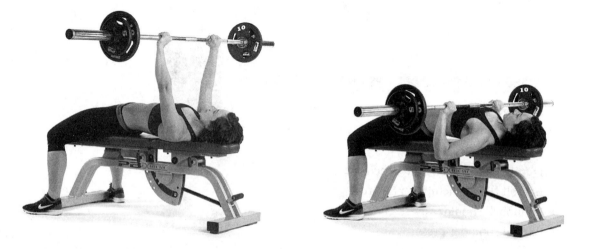

and your hands about one and a half times shoulder-width apart. Set your feet on the floor and wide apart, arch your back, pull your shoulder blades together, and tighten everything up, especially your grip. Lift the barbell off the supports or have a spotter lift the bar and hand it off to you. Hold it straight over your chest. *Pull the bar down* to the lower half of your chest, keeping your elbows close to your torso. Push back up to the starting position.

✳ Dumbbell Shoulder Press

THE SETUP: You just need a pair of dumbbells.

HOW TO DO IT: Stand holding the weights at the sides of your shoulders. Your palms can face in or out, whichever is more comfortable for you. Press the weights straight up over your shoulders, lower them, and repeat.

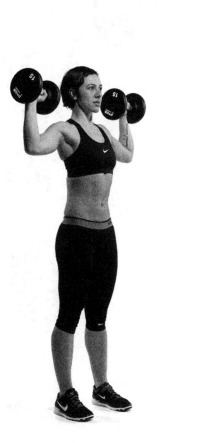
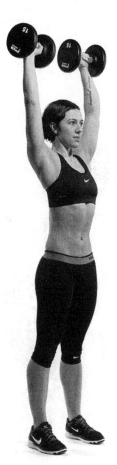

✳ Barbell Shoulder Press

THE SETUP: Set a barbell in the rack just below shoulder height—probably the same position you'd use for a front squat.

HOW TO DO IT: Grab the barbell overhand, your thumbs wrapped around it rather than even with your fingers. Now comes a tricky part: Slide your hands in or out until your forearms are perpendicular to the floor. (They'll probably be just slightly outside shoulder-width.) Tighten your grip and lift the bar off the supports, holding it at the top of your chest. Your elbows will be in front of your torso and beneath your wrists. Now for an even trickier part: *Press the bar straight up from your shoulders*, moving your head back just enough to avoid knocking yourself out. Finish with the weight over your shoulders and slightly behind your head with your arms straight. Lower it along the same path, once again ducking your head out of the way.

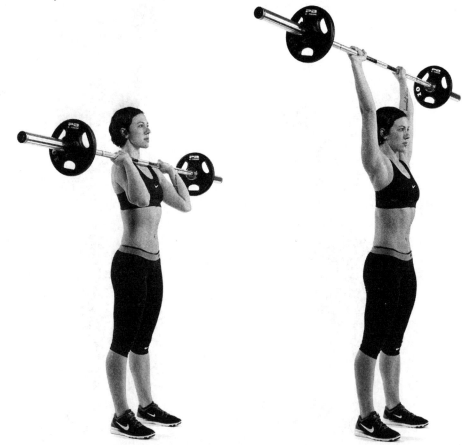

✴ Cable Chest Press

WHERE IT BECOMES AN OPTION: Phase Three, Stage 8, Workout B

WHAT IT DOES: I'm a big fan of exercises that accomplish multiple goals, as long as each goal is worth the effort and none of the goals cancels the others out. Doing a chest press on a Swiss ball, for example, adds a core-stability challenge while reducing work for your chest and shoulders. It's a win-lose exercise. But I see no downside to the standing chest press with a cable or bands. Your body is in a solid position to push as much weight as you can handle, and the heavier the weight, the more you'll feel it in your abdominal muscles, along with your chest, shoulders, and triceps. Another benefit, I think, is the break it offers your shoulder joints. Whatever press you choose for your main exercise in Phase Three—horizontal or vertical, with a barbell or dumbbells— you're going to impose some stress on your shoulders. You'll feel an immediate difference with cable and band presses.

THE SETUP: You can do the exercise with one or two arms at a time. Most of the time, in most gyms, you're better off using a single cable. The more crowded the gym is, the harder it'll be to tie up two cable machines. (Although that doesn't stop meatheads from doing it; at peak hours, it's the ultimate dick move.) Attach a D-shaped handle to one or both cables, and set it or them to chest height.

HOW TO DO IT

SINGLE CABLE: Grab the handle with your left hand and step forward, with your back to the machine, so you have tension in the cable. Get into a split stance with your right foot forward. Start with the handle next to your shoulder and your torso braced. Push it straight out while resisting any rotation from your hips and shoulders. Return to the starting position, do all your reps, then switch sides and repeat.

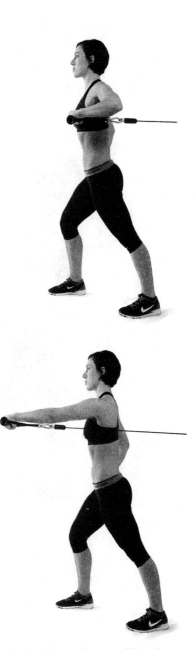

Note for the photos on this page and the next: Sometimes we don't realize we've made a mistake until we see them on the page. In this case, our model's body position is perfect, but the cable(s) should be over or alongside her arm(s), rather than underneath.

DUAL CABLES: Grab the handles and hold them at your shoulders. Get into a split stance with your right foot forward. Lean your entire body forward between 15 and 30 degrees, as if you're sprinting. Brace your torso. Push both handles straight out from your shoulders, and return to the starting position. For the next set, have your left foot forward.

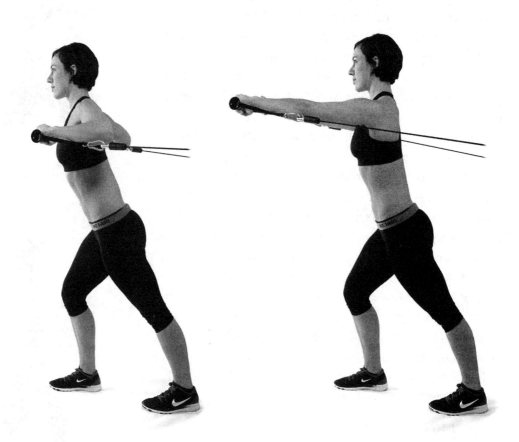

PULL

I've talked a lot so far about the role of the lats in supporting your back in exercises like deadlifts. Now you're going to use them the traditional way: as the vast swaths of muscle tissue that pull your arms back toward your torso when they're out in front of you, or extended overhead.

Same with your trapezius, the thick, diamond-shaped muscle that covers your upper and middle back and moves your shoulder blades up (a shrug), in (rowing), or down (climbing).

You may wonder why I just used *vast* and *thick*, which seem like pretty unappealing words when describing your physique. I'm thinking in relative terms. The latissimus dorsi, objectively, cover more real estate than any other muscle group. As for the trapezius, you don't want it to be small, at least not in proportion to your frame. Any action that requires moving or stabilizing your shoulder blades—which is to say, any meaningful human movement—depends on your traps. Think of an athlete whose physique you admire. It doesn't matter if it's a gymnast, golfer, ballerina, or CrossFitter; if you notice her, the odds are pretty good that she has great posture. And if she has great posture, she has a trapezius that's strong enough to pull her shoulder blades down and back, while just about every aspect of modern life conspires to pull them up and forward.

But for all their importance, pulling exercises are really simple. There are fewer exercises in this category than any other. You'll see lots of places in the program where Alwyn calls for a "chin-up, band-assisted chin-up, or lat pulldown." For higher reps, very few readers will be able to do chin-ups. That means you'll do a shitload of pulldowns. You'll want to use different variations in each stage, as described for each exercise.

✳ Dumbbell 3-Point Row

WHERE IT FIRST APPEARS: Phase One, Stage 1, Workout A

WHAT IT DOES: I flat-out love this exercise, along with its more challenging cousin, the dead-stop row, which you'll see in a moment. With your back in a safe position, supported above and below by one hand and both feet, you can work up to using a lot of weight without compromising your form.

THE SETUP: You need one dumbbell—the heaviest you can use for the reps Alwyn specifies—and a bench or box to rest your nonworking hand.

HOW TO DO IT: Grab the dumbbell and stand facing the box or bench. Bend forward at the hips and rest your nonworking hand on the bench. You want your back flat, knees bent, and the weight hanging straight down from your shoulder. Tighten everything so you have a solid, stable base. Pull the weight straight up to the side of your torso, lower it, finish all your reps, then switch hands and repeat the set.

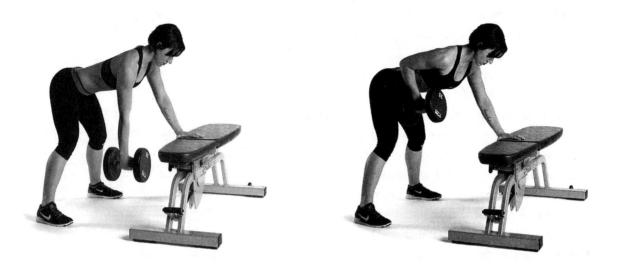

✳ Inverted Row

WHERE IT FIRST APPEARS: Phase One, Stage 1, Workout B

WHAT IT DOES: The inverted row is the opposite of a push-up in terms of muscle action, and only slightly less versatile. With experimentation and practice—and you'll have lots of opportunities for both—you can learn how to shift your grip and posture to hit your back and arm muscles in different ways. This may be the only exercise in which you can alter your form in the middle of a set. If you think you won't reach the rep target, you can bend your knees and move your heels closer to the bar, making it slightly easier but no less safe or effective.

THE SETUP: Set a barbell in a rack or Smith machine at a height that's appropriate for your current strength and the prescribed rep range. You'll want to set it higher (probably waist height or above) for lower strength and/or higher reps, and lower (hip height) if you're stronger and/or doing fewer reps.

HOW TO DO IT: Position yourself under the bar, looking up. Grab the bar overhand, with your hands about one and a half times shoulder-width—the same grip you'd use for a barbell bench press. Set your body in a straight line from neck to ankles as you hang with your arms straight. Pull your chest to the bar, return to the starting position, and repeat.

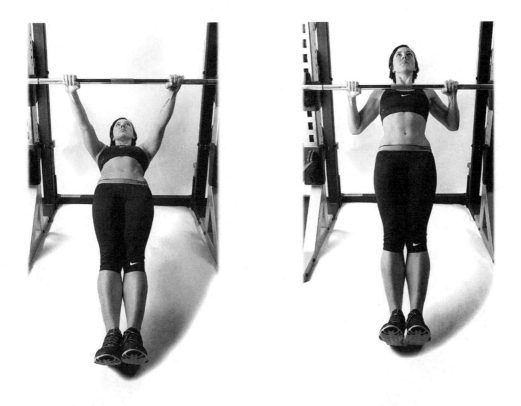

INVERTED ROW GRIP OPTIONS: With a *wide grip* (double shoulder-width), you'll pull the bar to your upper chest, with a shorter range of motion. It seems best for working your rear deltoids and the upper fibers of your trapezius while reducing the role of your lats. A *narrow grip* does the opposite: You'll pull to your lower chest, with a longer range of motion. An *underhand grip*, usually at or just inside shoulder-width, directly hits your biceps, which work in concert with your lats.

BADASS OPTIONS: At a certain point, you can't lower the bar any more and still hang from it with straight arms. To keep it challenging, you can *raise one foot in the air* to reduce your base of support. (Be sure to do half your reps with each foot off the ground.) Or you can set *your feet on a box or step*, which makes an inverted row even more inverted. Or you can *wear a weighted vest*.

✳ Suspended Row

WHERE IT BECOMES AN OPTION: Phase One, Stage 2, Workout A

WHAT IT DOES: You can use the suspended row in place of the inverted row at any point, starting with Stage 2. (Use the row as described for Stage 1, Special Workout, on p. 59.) As with the fixed-bar version, you can make it harder or easier by raising or lowering the handles of the suspension system.

THE SETUP: Set the straps of the suspension system to an appropriate height for your strength and the prescribed rep range.

HOW TO DO IT: Grab the handles and stand facing the attachment point. Walk back until, when you lean back on your heels, with your arms straight, your body is at a 45-degree angle to the floor. Align your body so it's straight from neck to ankles. Pull your body up and forward until the handles reach the sides of your torso. Lean back to return to the starting position, and repeat.

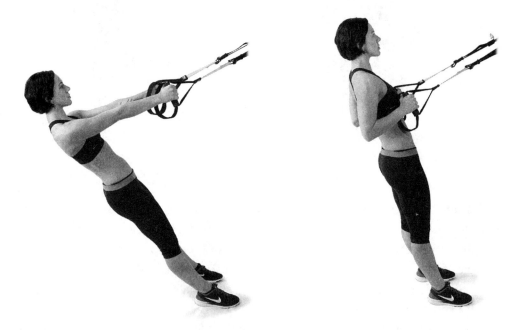

BADASS OPTION: The toughest variation is to set up with your chest directly beneath the attachment point of the straps. That is, the straps are perpendicular to the floor throughout the movement. In a study published in 2009, men doing that version with their knees bent and feet flat on the floor had more upper-back muscle activation than they did in two comparison exercises: the bent-over barbell row and standing single-arm cable row.

✳ Standing Single-Arm Cable Row

WHERE IT IS: Phase One, Stage 2, Workout B

WHAT IT DOES: The study mentioned in the badass option for the suspended row showed that the single-arm row is a really good way to work the lats. It's also a challenging antirotation exercise, in that you have to work hard to stabilize your core when pulling from one side at a time.

HOW TO DO IT: Attach a D-shaped handle to the cable and set it to waist height. Grab the handle and stand facing the machine with your arm straight, feet shoulder-width apart, and knees bent slightly. Tighten up your core. Pull the handle to the side of your waist, keeping your shoulders and hips square to the machine. Return to the starting position and repeat. Do all your reps, switch arms, and repeat.

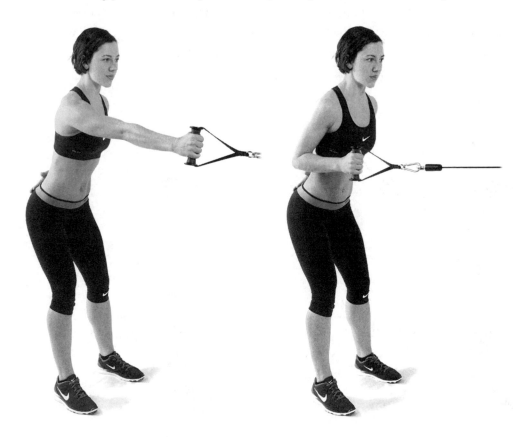

✳ Half-Kneeling X Pulldown

WHERE IT IS: Phase One, Stage 3, Workout A

WHAT IT DOES: This may be my favorite lat-pulldown variation. If you've never done it before, you'll feel it in your upper-back muscles the next day, a pretty good sign that it worked your traps and rear shoulders in a unique way.

THE SETUP: First you'll need dual cables. The easiest option: a lat-pulldown machine that has two cables attached to a single weight stack. A lot of gyms now have them, and some companies even make them for the home-gym market. The second-best choice is two cables attached to separate weight stacks. It could be a cable-crossover station or two machines right next to each other. (As I mentioned with the cable chest press, in a crowded gym it's hard to use two cable stations simultaneously.) In either case, set the pulleys at the highest position, and attach D-shaped handles to both cables.

HOW TO DO IT: Grab the handles with your opposite-side hands and position yourself on one knee in between the two. In the starting position, one forearm will be over the other, forming the letter X. Pull the handles diagonally until your hands reach the front of your shoulders—right hand at right shoulder, left at left. Return to the starting position and repeat. Switch legs for the next set.

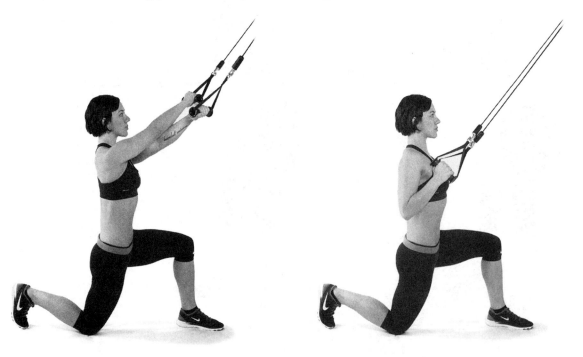

✳ Dumbbell Single-Arm Dead-Stop Row

WHERE IT IS: Phase One, Stage 3, Workout B

WHAT IT DOES: With the weight starting on the floor each rep, the dead-stop row is a total-body exercise, with all the challenges that go along with it. You'll need a strong brace with your core muscles to prevent rotating at the hips and lower back, and as you get tired it'll be increasingly difficult to avoid lifting your torso to help you keep the weight moving.

THE SETUP: You need one dumbbell—the heaviest you can use—and a bench or box to rest your nonworking hand. Set the dumbbell on the floor next to the box or bench.

HOW TO DO IT: Position yourself with your nonworking hand on the bench and the weight beneath the shoulder of your working arm. Spread your feet wide and bend your knees to get your torso low enough for you to grab the weight. With your back flat and tightly braced, pull the weight to the side of your torso. Lower it to the floor. Reset your body. Do all your reps, then switch sides and repeat.

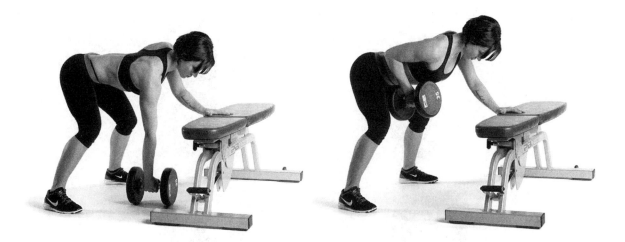

✳ Lat Pulldown

WHERE IT BECOMES AN OPTION: Phase Two, Stage 4, Workout A

WHAT IT DOES: Thanks to the nearly vertical range of motion, the pulldown does a bang-up job working your lats—exactly what you expect. Interestingly, muscle activation doesn't change all that much when you change the width of your grip. One study with experienced lifters found the lats and biceps did about the same amount of work with wide, medium, or narrow overhand grips. However, when you shift to a narrow, underhand grip, you'll work your biceps harder and your lats a bit less. Here you'll start with the most common grip—medium-width, overhand. It's up to you to adjust your grip in subsequent programs.

THE SETUP: Attach a long bar to a high cable.

HOW TO DO IT: Grab the bar overhand, your hands about one and a half times shoulder-width apart. Kneel in front of the weight stack, pulling the bar down with you but keeping your arms straight. Straighten your torso and tighten your core.

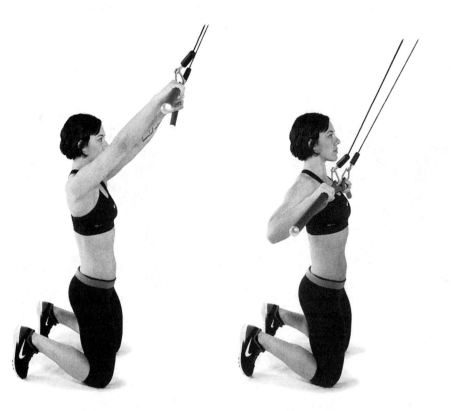

Pull the bar down to your upper chest. Finish the movement by *pushing your chest out to meet the bar*. Return to the starting position and repeat.

HOW TO DO IT BETTER: Inexperienced lifters tend to make the pulldown an arm exercise, activating their biceps at the expense of their lats. (Complete beginners often do something even worse: they pull the bar down the front of the torso by internally rotating their upper arms.) But a study published in 2009 found that when novice female lifters were told how to activate their lat muscles, they were able to make them work harder, without actually reducing the amount of work done by their biceps. The secret? Focusing on the targeted muscles as they work, what bodybuilders call the mind–muscle connection.

PULLDOWN OPTIONS

* Kneel on one knee, instead of both.
* Change attachments for different programs and different rep ranges (you can probably use the heaviest weights with the triangle attachment, the one in which your palms are turned toward each other and several inches apart).
* Try it standing, with one foot on the seat of the pulldown station to keep you balanced.

✴ Chin-Up

WHERE IT BECOMES AN OPTION: Phase Two, Stage 4, Workout A

WHAT IT DOES: Most of the time, if you can do chin-ups instead of pulldowns for the same number of reps, you should. It's a much more challenging exercise, and not just because you're lifting your entire body weight instead of a fraction of it. With your body dangling from the bar, you'll employ more stabilizing muscles.

THE SETUP: You just need a bar high enough and solid enough to support your full weight.

HOW TO DO IT: Grab the bar with a shoulder-width, underhand grip, and hang with your arms straight, knees bent slightly, and feet crossed behind you. Pull your chest up to the bar, lower yourself, and repeat.

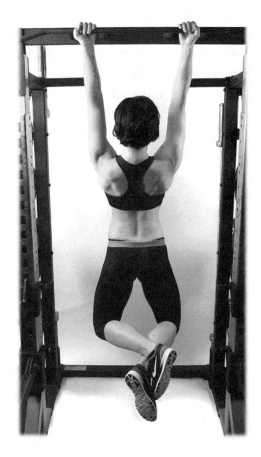

CHIN-UP OPTIONS

As a skinny teenager, I regularly did sets of up to 15 pull-ups—the version with a slightly wider, overhand grip. Today, a single pull-up feels like sticking a knife into my shoulder. I can do chin-ups without pain, but I struggle to remember the last time I reached double digits. So I'm in awe of any woman who can use the chin-up for the prescribed reps in any of Alwyn's programs. Here's what to do if you can't:

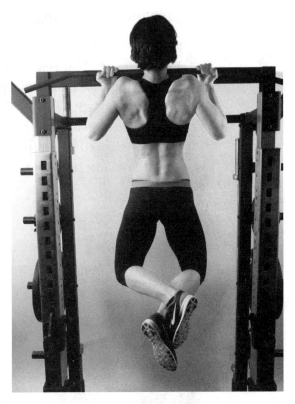

DO FEWER REPS: Suppose a workout calls for 3 sets of 10 reps. And suppose you can only do 5 chin-ups per set. You'll probably get a better workout by doing sets of 5 chin-ups vs. 10 lat pulldowns, especially if you increase your strength enough to add 1 or 2 reps.

USE A BAND FOR ASSISTANCE: Attach a resistance band to the chin-up bar, and loop it around your knees or feet. The band will help you get started from the bottom position.

USE A TRAINING PARTNER: Some lifters get stuck in the middle of the lift, rather than the bottom. The band doesn't help you through that sticking point. If you have a training partner, you can have her push you up to complete each rep. In my experience, it's best to boost from the ankles.

START FROM THE FLOOR: There's no rule that says a chin-up has to start from a dead hang. You can set a barbell in the squat rack so it allows you to stand or kneel on the floor with your arms fully extended overhead. Pull yourself up from that position.

✳ Standing Single-Arm Low-Cable Row

WHERE IT IS: Phase Two, Stage 4, Workout B

WHAT IT DOES: This is a small variation on the single-arm row described on p. 225, using the same muscles but pulling from a lower angle.

THE SETUP: Attach a D-shaped handle to a low cable.

HOW TO DO IT: Grab the handle with one hand, and stand facing the cable machine as described earlier, only with your torso bent farther forward from the hips. Pull the handle to the outside of your hip. Do all your reps, switch sides, and repeat.

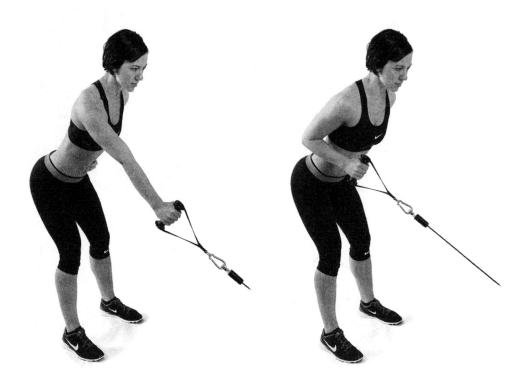

✳ Cable Bent-Over Row (Dual Handles)

WHERE IT IS: Phase Two, Stage 5, Workout A

WHAT IT DOES: This works the same muscles as the other cable rows, only with both sides working together. You should be able to use a lot more weight, and if you focus on the working muscles, you can feel strong contractions in your middle and lower traps, along with your lats.

THE SETUP: Three ways to do it: You can attach two D-shaped handles to a single cable, with the pulley at the lowest setting; use a rope, with the attachment ring in the middle; or use two cables, with both pulleys in the bottommost position.

HOW TO DO IT: Same as the other rows, only with the handles in both hands and both arms extended in front of you. Pull the handles to the sides of your waist, return to the starting position, and repeat.

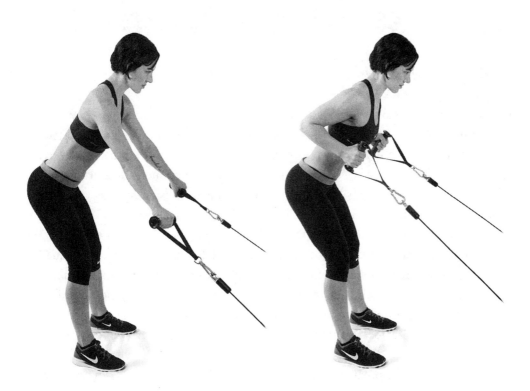

Intervals, Cardio, and the Perils of All of the Above

THE WORKOUTS IN *STRONG* EMPHASIZE A lot more than pure strength, as of course you know by now. Alwyn's goal is to give you a complete fitness program, based on the very real possibility that two or three of his workouts may be the only exercise you get in a typical week. So the program includes components to improve every aspect of fitness, starting with mobility and movement skills and ending with a furious 10 minutes of interval training.

But even though each part of the workout is neatly delineated on your training log, and in the chapters of our book, nobody can tell you where one fitness quality begins and another ends. Someone who's completely new to all this will probably get stronger from the mobility and core exercises because they use muscles in unfamiliar ways. Strength training often increases mobility, and sometimes even improves cardiovascular fitness. And intervals have been shown to offer two extraordinary benefits.

First among them: fat loss. Intervals, because they take a lot of effort and focus, generate a lot of adrenaline—much more than steady-pace endurance exercise, which burns more overall calories. Adrenaline releases fat from storage and allows your body to burn more of it. The hormone remains elevated after you finish your work-out, as does your heart rate. So you're burning more calories (because of the higher heart rate) and continuing to release more fat from your cells (thanks to the adrenaline). It's also possible—and maybe even likely—that your appetite will be temporarily suppressed following your workout.

Then there's the long-term benefit of increased aerobic fitness. Interval-training studies lasting 12 weeks or more typically show double-digit-percentage improve-ments in VO_2max, a measure of your maximum oxygen consumption relative to your body size.

No matter how you choose to do the intervals in Phase One and Phase Two, the goal is to work hard for the amount of time Alwyn designates, or until your heart rate reaches a predetermined maximum. Then you recover, as described in Chapters 6 and 7. Your options include the following:

Outdoors
- Run
- Cycle
- Climb stairs

Indoor Cardio Machines
- Treadmill
- Stationary bike
- Elliptical
- Rowing machine
- Stairclimber/Jacob's ladder

Other Gym Equipment
- Push and/or pull a sled (shown on the next page)
- Loaded carries (shown on the following pages)
- Punch and/or kick a heavy bag
- Jump rope
- Use battling ropes, with one or both arms
- Swing a kettlebell (shown on p. 184)

No Space, No Equipment

- Shadow box
- Jumping jacks
- Calisthenics

✳ Sled Push/Pull

If you have a sled and the space to use it, you can push or pull until you reach your target for time or heart rate. You can load the sled up with weights, push slowly, and use it as an accessory strength exercise while also getting the benefits of metabolic training. Or you can go light and push faster. For pulling, if your gym has a harness designed for sled dragging (or if you can afford to buy one for home use), that should be your first choice. For our photos, we combined a TRX with a strap from another piece of equipment, which works well enough to use in my own workouts.

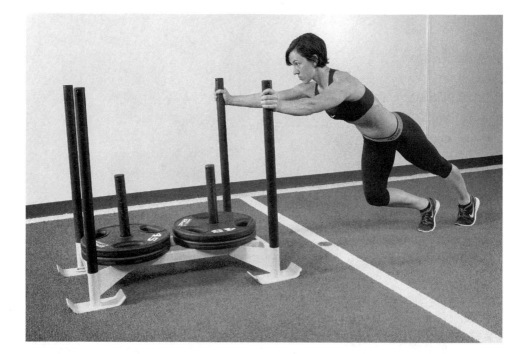

✴ Loaded Carries

Execution is simple: Pick up something heavy, and carry it back and forth until you reach your target time or heart rate. Your options include the following:

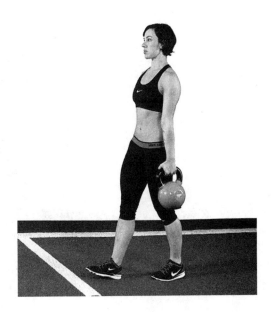

- Suitcase: carry one dumbbell or kettlebell, or even a barbell, at arm's length at your side; you can alternate sides, or switch halfway through an interval.
- Farmer's: carry two dumbbells, kettlebells, or barbells at your sides.
- Waiter's: carry one or two dumbbells or kettlebells overhead; you can also use a barbell, weight plate, or sandbag.

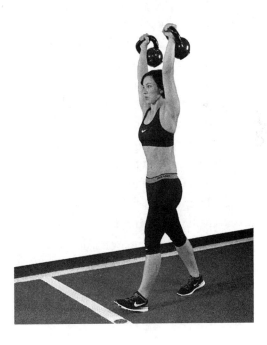

- Bear hug: hold a weight plate or sandbag against your chest.

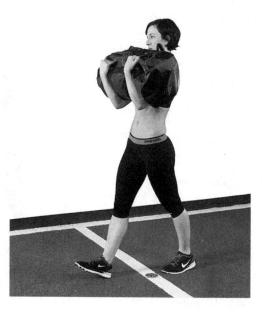

- Shoulder: hold one or two kettlebells in the rack position, or a slosh pipe (a length of PVC pipe filled with water and plugged at the ends) in the front squat or bear hug position.

Many of the choices in these lists—which are by no means exhaustive—do more than crank up your heart rate. Sled pushes, for example, can be a great muscle-building exercise for your entire lower body. (They may be the best calf-targeting option in the entire program.) Carries can improve grip strength, core stability, posture, and arm and shoulder development. Swings can perk up the frowniest of glutes.

In fact, there's so much you can accomplish in the final 10 minutes of your workouts that you may find yourself asking a question I hear a lot from readers, and Alwyn probably hears every day: If some interval training is good, wouldn't more be even better?

The answer is a lot more complicated than you'd expect.

WHEN TO SAY WHEN

Let's revisit something we mentioned in Chapter 2: We know beyond any doubt that moving is better than sitting. When you compare those who sit more with those who move more, the movers are less likely to have diabetes or cardiovascular disease, or to die prematurely. The research specific to sitting is relatively new, which is why it's gotten so much attention the past few years. But for as long as I've been writing about exercise, we've known that people who go from doing nothing to doing something get the biggest health benefits. It doesn't seem to matter what the something is.

Once you're up and moving, it makes sense to focus on specific goals. Again, it doesn't seem to matter all that much which ones. As long as whatever you do is challenging enough to move you from the lowest to the second-lowest categories of cardiovascular fitness, you'll get a significant benefit. Additional health benefits accrue in a more or less linear way from there.

But the kind of benefits you seek when you commit to a program like Alwyn's— visible, measurable improvements in strength, athleticism, and appearance—come only with serious exercise, with consistently pushing yourself out of your comfort zone. You're training your body to do more, and to do it better.

The training process works like this:

1. You challenge your body with a training stimulus.
2. You allow your body to recover from that challenge.
3. Your body adapts to the stimulus by getting stronger or faster or leaner or better conditioned.
4. You apply your newfound strength or speed or endurance.

Alwyn's program gives you the stimulus, with heavy lifting and short but intense intervals three times a week. But step 2 is on you, and it's tricky. You can't get to steps 3 and 4 with inadequate or incomplete recovery. The balance between stimulus and recovery will be different for each of us. Even at the individual level, it'll always be a moving target. You can do more when the stress of your everyday life is manageable but less when you're dealing with crises at home or work.

That doesn't mean you shouldn't do anything outside of Alwyn's program. You should. Doing light physical activity—a daily walk, for example—can lead to better recovery and better overall results. It makes sense to assume that yoga or Pilates classes could also be good choices for nonlifting days.

For many of you, though, that won't be enough. Some will want to combine Alwyn's workouts with endurance training, and I'll talk about that in the next section. Others will combine them with training for a specific sport or favorite activity. We love sports and would never try to talk you out of it. But if you're pursuing something extra because you think it will accelerate or somehow improve your results, we suggest reading this quote from strength coach Alexander Cortes: "There is this idea that if training is 'good,' or going well, that by adding more to it, it will become 'great.' This tends to make things go from good to shit really fast."

To which Alwyn adds: "I can put anything I want in these workouts. I can write a two-a-day, seven-days-a-week program. If I felt more was better, I would've put more into them. The bottom line is that all movement is likely to be helpful, with this caveat: If it negatively impacts your ability to train hard in the next workout, it's a bad idea."

So now let's talk about endurance training.

CARDIO CONSIDERATIONS

When you lift, you ask your body to remodel itself in a specific way, making muscle fibers bigger and stronger. But success in an endurance sport requires a different and potentially conflicting set of adaptations, making muscle cells more efficient at providing oxygen and nutrients.

If you're tempted to try it, you're hardly alone. Athletes and fitness buffs have been trying to find a balance between the two for as long as humans have engaged in systematic exercise. Researchers call it *concurrent training* and have studied the potential interference effect extensively.

Some things we've learned from that research:

- Cardio exercise probably won't affect your upper-body strength and muscle development. But it can have a big effect on lower-body strength and size.
- Running interferes more with lower-body muscle than does cycling. Both running and lifting create muscle damage, and the combination may prevent full recovery from either one.
- That said, the combination of running and lifting is, on average, better for fat loss. Lifting plus cycling produces no better results than lifting without cycling.

- Cycling, however, may enhance muscle growth. That's the conclusion of a series of studies by Swedish researchers, who had volunteers do a combination of lifting and cycling with one leg while only lifting with the other. After five weeks, the quadriceps of the cross-trained leg showed more growth.
- The more endurance exercise you do, the bigger the interference effect, especially on strength. The decline is almost linear for each additional day of cardio. (It's not at all linear for muscle growth. In at least one meta-analysis, four days a week looks much worse than either three or five.)
- The results are similar when you look at minutes per day of cardio. Longer daily sessions create more interference than shorter ones for both strength and muscle development.

That's as much as we can learn from research, which, it's worth noting, was conducted with subjects who may not resemble you. They may have been older, younger, leaner, heavier, or less female. They may have more or less experience or genetic predispositions that make them more or less adaptable to the type of training the researchers had them do.

And there's one more key difference, as Alwyn points out: "Those studies were based on traditional strength training—typically machines, straight sets, long rest periods. That doesn't reflect the type of training our readers are doing. These are full-body workouts with full-body exercises in multiple planes of movement. It's a different stimulus from what researchers consider 'strength training.'"

MIX 'EM, MATCH 'EM . . .

In trying to figure out what works best for you, you'll probably start with what *has* worked. Past performance certainly can tell you two important things:

- What you like to do
- What your body does well

What you may not know: Will the body you have *now* adapt as well to those activities as it did in the past? Can you recover adequately from multiple types of exercise? If the past was two pregnancies ago, or premenopause, or before you got promoted into a position that requires longer hours and/or more travel, you really don't know until you try.

A few guidelines:

If you're eating less with the goal of losing weight: Food is energy, as we discussed in Chapter 3, and it's illogical to expect your body to produce substantially more movement with less fuel. Alwyn's workouts are stressful to a well-fueled body. In an energy deficit, full recovery becomes a challenge. You want to avoid any additional type of training that could compromise it. But a daily walk, as aforementioned, should help with recovery while also burning a few extra calories. You aren't going for speed or distance or any other performance measure. Your only goal is to spend more time on your feet without putting additional stress on your muscles or joints.

If your primary goal is pure strength: I asked Greg Nuckols, a record-setting powerlifter, how much cardio competitive lifters do, and what types. He asked if I wanted to know what they *should* do or what they *actually* do. The latter, I replied. He said it's all over the place. He mentioned a powerlifter who trains as a rower in his off-season and another who jogs several times a week, except in the immediate run-up to a contest. At the opposite extreme are powerlifters who don't do any conditioning outside of the weight room.

Eric Cressey, a former competitive powerlifter who currently specializes in training baseball players, recommends staying out of the "no-man's-land" of medium-intensity, medium-speed endurance work. He believes strength athletes do best with low-intensity cardio several times a week—even if it's as simple and easy as walking on a treadmill—with perhaps one session a week of all-out sprints: run hard for 10 seconds, and recover for up to 2 or 3 minutes.

Keep in mind that pure strength is a singular goal. Simultaneously training for endurance, hypertrophy, or low body fat will compromise your results. But it's not a goal you have to train for year-round. Four to six months a year of dedicated max-strength work might give you exactly what you want, with less risk of injury or burnout. Focus on something else the rest of the year, while maintaining a base of strength.

If your primary goal is endurance performance: I've heard from several readers over the years who told me they ran faster after incorporating Alwyn's NROL programs, despite lower mileage in training. It's a good reminder that human physiology resists specialization. A stronger body can almost always do more than a weaker one.

That said, if running or cycling or swimming long distances is your *main* goal, you have to prioritize those adaptations in your training. Two strength workouts a week should be plenty. Stick with Phase One and Phase Two; the Phase Three work-outs require more recovery and would be more likely to compromise results from your sport-specific workouts. If you're doing speed work while training for a race, you may want to skip the intervals.

If your primary goal is to achieve low body fat: Now we get to the biggest reason most readers pick up a book like *Strong*: You want to look better than you do now. Women at the front end of the process often equate progress with a dress size or a number on the scale. That way lies madness, as quite a few of you have described to me. The scale doesn't know what you look like, much less how strong you are or how good you feel. It's just a number detached from context.

Those of you who commit to a program like this one understand the value of getting stronger, of developing metabolically powerful muscle, and of using that muscle to become leaner over time. Many of you also understand how frustrating the process can be. There's never a straight line connecting effort to results. Just as no one can tell you exactly what or how much to eat to achieve your goals, neither can anyone prescribe the perfect mix of exercise inside and outside the weight room.

Just about anything works the first few times you try it. But then your body adapts. There's a limit to how much volume you can add before it interferes with recovery or you get hurt. Worse is the feeling that you're being pulled in multiple directions. When you lift, you're frustrated that you aren't stronger. When you go for a run the next day, you're frustrated that you can't run farther or faster. When you try on clothes, you're frustrated when the dress that looks perfect on the rack is too small for your hips or thighs or waist.

I love this description of the dilemma from Lisa Lilge, who manages an NROL-focused group on Facebook: "We have a bad habit of chasing too many rabbits at once."

Her *we* referred to women, but these days I encounter just as much rabbit-chasing from men: "I'm 6 foot 2, 120 pounds. My goal is to add 30 pounds of solid muscle. But I don't want to lose my abs. And I want to do it entirely with body-weight exercises. And I want to use intermittent fasting." I'm exaggerating, but not as much as you think. All the concerns are real. They just happened to come from different readers. Guys will watch *300* on cable and decide they want to be both big and ripped, like those Spartan warriors who for some reason went to battle in capes and Speedos. They'll see an ad from someone selling a body-weight-only training program and decide that's the best way to look like one of the guys in *300*, even though the actors trained with weights. Or they'll decide that long periods of self-starvation are the key to just about any goal because they read a blog post from someone with an undiagnosed eating disorder.

Here's Alwyn's hierarchy of training priorities, based on your ambition and available time to train:

Three days a week: You're good to go with the programs in *Strong*.

Four days a week: "This is where it starts to get interesting," Alwyn says. You could add a day of intervals to three *Strong* workouts. Or you could try two strength workouts plus two days of interval training, 20 to 30 minutes per session. Alwyn and his trainers have been testing this system with clients who're primarily interested in fat loss and are encouraged by the early results.

Five days a week: This one's easy to prescribe, less easy to perform: Three *Strong* workouts plus two days of intervals, probably 20 minutes' worth on both days.

Six days a week: If the five-day prescription isn't enough, Alwyn says your sixth workout should be one focused on recovery: mobility exercises (like those in RAMP) with foam rolling and perhaps some stretches; low-intensity cardio (walk-jog, not a serious run); or perhaps a long hike.

But on the seventh day: "I like one full rest day per week, with no exercise," Alwyn says. "I'm okay with going for a walk or a hike. The dog needs to get outside, after all. But the key to all this is to avoid anything that makes you sore or fatigued, or does anything to prevent you from setting records in the weight room."

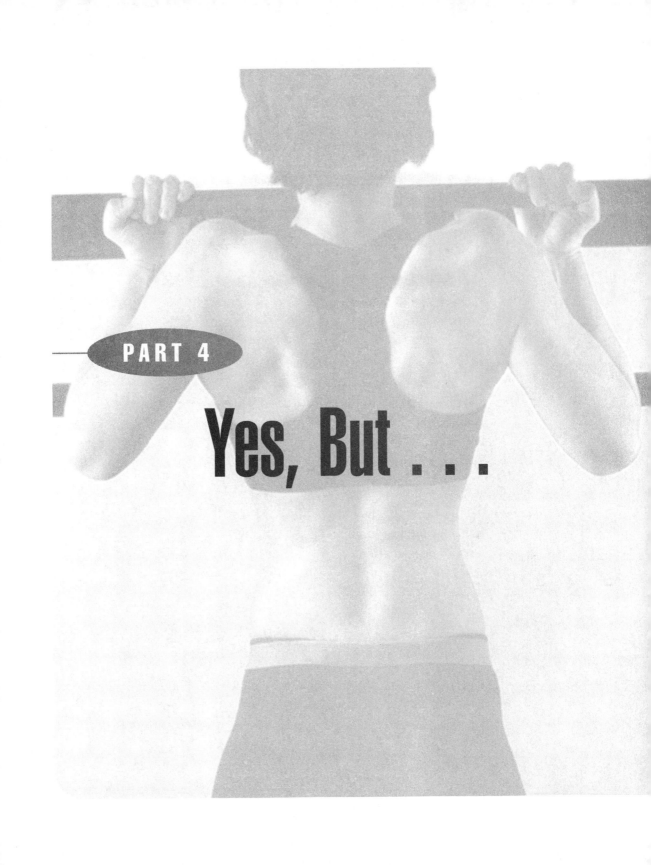

PART 4

Yes, But . . .

All Those
Nagging Doubts

I'VE WRITTEN A LOT OF WORKOUT books, which means I've written a lot of final chapters of workout books (along with opening chapters, and everything in between). Each time I try my best to head off the questions I'm pretty sure you'll want to ask. And each time I'm surprised. Your questions are never what I expected.

That's why, for the first time, I asked readers what they wanted Alwyn and me to address in *Strong* before I started writing. I thought it would liberate me from some of the anxiety that builds when I spend a year or two on a book without really knowing whether it's going to satisfy the audience. Many of you answered. And it only made the anxiety worse.

I'm not saying it wasn't helpful. It was. You told me you wanted more information about how to swap exercises in or out. I'm pretty sure *Strong* has more options than any of our five previous books (and more than *NROL for Women* and the original *NROL* combined). You said you wanted to know more about how to make progress. If you're willing to read closely, you'll see specific tips throughout the exercise chapters. And when you said you wanted more information about how to combine

Alwyn's programs with other types of training, we made that the focus of an entire chapter.

But here's what worries me: A lot of the requests were *extremely* specific.

Take this comment, which I'm only lightly paraphrasing: "Women want more information about how to lose fat after pregnancy. They want ripped abs, too, and a rehash of *NROL for Women* won't do. They want relatable, easy-to-follow programs that get results."

Let's take them one at a time:

Fat loss after pregnancy: Everyone with Internet access has seen pictures of women who rock perfect six-packs an hour after dropping triplets. The story they tell is one I've heard from models and fitness professionals more times than I can count: "My body is the result of sacrifice, discipline, and hard work. Only weak people make excuses." I don't doubt that they have the motivation and work ethic. But they also have an extraordinarily rare genetic makeup that allows them to recover quickly and do challenging workouts immediately after childbirth. All we can advise women with certainty is to proceed with caution, because a postpregnancy body is vulnerable and easily injured. Do what your body allows, and for the love of all that's good in the world, pay attention to the signals it sends. If the signals are all green lights, have at it. If you get a flashing red, hit the brakes.

Ripped abs: That's a bodybuilding program—a minimum of five days a week in the gym, daily cardio during contest prep, and a diet with no margin for error. We have a lot of respect for what bodybuilders do. But it's not what Alwyn does with his clients, or what either of us promises to our readers.

Rehash of *NROL for Women*: This is our fourth book post-*Women*. No reasonable person would call any of them a rehash of our most popular title.

Relatable, easy-to-follow programs that get results: You can have an easy-to-follow program, or one that gets results for lifters at all levels. Not both. As for "relatable," if it means "realistic," we think we delivered. If it means, "I'm going to like every part of it," you'll be disappointed. Because after a lifetime of lifting, I can promise you this: If you enjoy every aspect of your training program, you aren't pushing yourself hard enough to get results.

Lots of other comments raised lots of specific concerns. Menopause, for example. I've watched my wife go through it, and I wouldn't wish those hot flashes and unpredictable moods on anybody. But I'll be damned if I know of any training program that specifically addresses the physiological changes that follow. When I asked Alwyn, all he could suggest is that menopause-related sleep disturbances can interfere with recovery. Otherwise, training is training. To misquote a former government official, you go to the gym with the body you have, not the body you might want or wish to have at a later time.

Which is a perfect segue to this.

YOUR BODY, YOUR PROGRAM, YOUR CHOICE

The book you've almost finished reading includes nine total-body workout programs, each of which will take about a month to complete. Most of you will be able to do each stage at least twice and still see substantial gains. Which means, for most readers, this is a program you can do for as long as you're interested in continuing.

Is it tailored to your individual needs and interests? Absolutely not. But that's the genius of it. Alwyn and his coaches at Results Fitness use this template with almost every client, from complete beginners who've never felt the cold, indifferent steel of a barbell in their palms to elite amateur and professional athletes.

Some of the novices assume they aren't capable of doing this type of training. Until they try it and realize they can. But you know what's interesting? No advanced athlete has ever told Alwyn these workouts were too basic or easy for her. There's a simple reason: The more experience you have, the more challenging the program becomes.

You know how I know? Because I've been working out for more than 40 years, *and these workouts kicked my ass.* There were multiple times, starting with the very first workouts in Phase One, when I overdid things and ended up sore for the next two days. And did I mention that I'm a guy? True story. I've got the male-pattern baldness to prove it. I even cry during war movies.

That said, no system is perfect for every lifter. *Strong* is about building strength as part of a total package, one that includes movement quality, muscle development, and cardiovascular fitness. It's not a bodybuilding or powerlifting program. Nor is it ideal for someone with serious health issues or recovering from injuries that limit your ability to do basic exercises. If your primary goal is to train for a specific sport like a triathlon, you'll do best with a program written for triathletes, saving these workouts for your off-season. It's not a body-weight-only program, and there is no DVD or app.

Strong is for everyone else, which is to say women who want to lift, who have access to basic strength-training equipment, and who are comfortable being occasionally uncomfortable—lifting heavy things, learning new exercises, testing the limits of antiperspirant technology. And if you're afflicted with resting bitch face when you *aren't* straining, you sure don't want to look in a mirror when you're attempting a new personal record on the deadlift.

It's for that instant, when you do something you haven't done before, something you didn't think you *could* do at this moment in your life, that Alwyn and I wrote *Strong*. We didn't write it for everybody. Question is, Did we write it for you?

A Beginner's Guide to Lifting

IF YOU CAN MOVE, YOU CAN lift. Take away all the jargon and buzzwords and abbreviations and complicated instructions, and strength training is simply a way to improve on what your body does naturally. You already know how to push, pull, bend, squat, stride, and turn. The next step is to learn a series of exercises based on those natural movements—which, ironically, will sometimes seem completely *un*natural.

At those moments, take comfort in knowing that every successful lifter started just like you, with no idea what he or she was doing. I once asked Dave Draper, one of the most famous bodybuilders of the 1960s (and the first whose name I knew and remembered), what he did to get started. He said he did what everyone did back then: He got a set of weights and a couple of charts that he taped to the wall. And then he lifted. He did the exercises on the charts, and if he wasn't satisfied with his results, he sometimes "invented" exercises to fill in the gaps. Those exercises already existed, but without a training manual or coach, there was no way for him to know.

You, on the other hand, have a training manual, and a possibly infinite number of potential coaches. The Internet gives you access to both coauthors, and on social media you can connect with lots of your fellow lifters, including many who started with *The New Rules of Lifting for Women* and will be happy to help you with *Strong*.

The Lingo

Sets and reps are the basic units of strength training. Rep, short for repetition, means a single execution of an exercise. One push-up = 1 rep. A set is a series of consecutive repetitions. So 5 push-ups = 1 set of 5, which is sometimes abbreviated as 1 × 5.

With most exercises, you'll do multiple sets, with a rest in between. You'll also alternate between two or more exercises, which is fully explained in Chapter 7.

A workout is the completion of all the sets and reps of all the exercises Alwyn specifies. In a typical workout, you'll do perhaps 20 different exercises. It should take 50 to 60 minutes.

About half those exercises are included in the warm-up, which Alwyn calls RAMP, which stands for range of motion, activation of muscles, and movement preparation and is explained in detail in Chapter 11. The goal is to get your body warm, limber, and ready for bigger challenges.

Next you'll do one, two, or sometimes three exercises for your *core*, which are detailed in Chapter 12. We define the core as all the muscles that help stabilize your lower back and pelvis. Most workout programs, including the one in *NROL for Women*, put these exercises at the end of each training session. But starting with our third book, *NROL for Abs*, Alwyn moved them to the beginning of our programs, to emphasize the importance of a strong, stable core. (If you're wondering why we don't include familiar exercises like crunches, you'll find the full explanation in *Abs*.)

That brings you to the *strength* exercises, covered in Chapters 13 and 14. There are usually two pairs, which means four altogether. The goal, obviously, is to get stronger from one workout to the next in each exercise.

The final part of each workout is some type of *interval training*, which is introduced in Chapter 7, with some specific options listed in Chapter 15. You go as hard as you can, then rest, for the time Alwyn specifies. It'll change from workout to workout.

There are usually two workouts per stage, labeled as Workout A and Workout B. Remember that each workout is a complete training session, which requires at least 48 hours of recovery. The system is explained in full in Chapter 6.

Gym Etiquette

No matter how well you understand manners and civility in the Emily Post sense of the words, you probably won't figure out the peculiar etiquette of health clubs until you've violated one of the many unwritten rules. A stranger will give you a dirty look, an exaggerated sigh of frustration, or perhaps even a verbal rebuke. Even if the stranger sees that you're new to the milieu (no matter how hard you try to hide it, it's usually obvious) and tries to explain your mistake in a friendly way, you may misinterpret both the message and its intent.

I'll give you a specific example:

I used to belong to a gym that was owned by an orthopedic practice. It was a great gym, the best I ever got to use on a daily basis until I switched to an even better one, where we shot the photos in this book. But it also had more older, inexperienced lifters than I'd ever seen in one place. Many of them, I'd wager, had never seen a weight room, much less trained in one. Now they were working out next to bodybuilders, powerlifters, and lifelong gym rats like me. It made for some awkward moments.

One time, when I needed to use a bench, I noticed that all but two were occupied. Those two were blocked by a woman standing between them while doing lateral raises, an exercise in which you lift dumbbells out to your sides. "Don't block equipment you aren't using" is one of the fundamental rules of gym etiquette. But I figured, correctly, that she had no idea of the rule or how she stood in violation of it.

"Ma'am," I said while she was in between sets, "could you please stand back here to do that exercise?"

She turned and hit me with a look cold enough to freeze a volcano. "Why's that?"

"Because that way you won't block those two benches."

She looked at the benches, looked at me, and turned and stalked out of the weight room. I found out later that she complained to a manager about being harassed. I never saw her again, which is just as well. Someone who's wound up that tight has no business in a room filled with potentially lethal blunt objects.

Weight-room etiquette can be summed up in a few sentences:

1. Don't block or set your towel and water bottle on equipment you aren't using.
2. Don't sit on equipment in between sets.
3. Put things away after you use them.
4. Wipe your perspiration off pads and benches.

In my experience, beginners are really good at the last two but utterly clueless about the others. Like I said, it's not obvious, and if no one tells you, how would you know?

The bigger problems I see relate to safety. If you don't know what to watch out for, there's a chance you'll put yourself or someone else at needless risk. Read on for a few pointers.

Give Lifters Space

Longtime lifters understand the geometry of the weight room. It's sort of like a checkerboard, but based on rectangles instead of squares. You have to give people space to move forward or back, or to lift a weight to the side. Never stand right next to someone who's lifting. And never, ever cross in front of someone who's in the middle of a set unless there's no other way to get around her. It breaks her concentration.

Respect the Mirror

Weird as it seems, lifters often pick their spots based on how well they can see themselves in a mirror. Cutting off someone's angle to the mirror is kind of like cutting off someone in traffic. Unless you have a really good reason, it's a rude and hostile thing to do.

Pay Attention!

I may be the last gym rat in the world who doesn't use an iPod in the weight room. It's not because I enjoy the music on the gym's sound system; I rarely do. But if I'm forced to choose between music I don't like and not using one of my five senses, it's an easy choice for me.

In my view, a lifter who can't hear what's going on around her is like a driver who doesn't use a turn signal because she's talking on her cell phone. She can't hear when you ask if you can work in on a piece of equipment or when you say "excuse me" because she's in your path.

The gym is a dangerous place only if you're not paying attention. To pay attention, you need to open your eyes and your ears. I understand why weight room veterans want to hear their own music and separate themselves from the often-mindless chatter of the less serious lifters. But when beginners cut themselves off, they assume a risk that simply isn't worth taking.

Appendix B
Strength-Training Equipment

ALWYN'S WORKOUTS REQUIRE BASIC STRENGTH-TRAINING equipment, which I'll explain in this section. You can either join a gym that has what you need or buy it for your home. (I'll give you specific tips as we go along.) Over the years our readers have had success with both choices. What *won't* work: radically modifying the program so you can do it with minimal equipment or with no equipment at all.

We've heard every argument and excuse. We know some people don't like working out in health clubs or can't afford one or don't have convenient access. We know many people who train at home can't afford or find room for all the stuff they need. We sympathize, but we can't change the parameters of Alwyn's training system without changing the system itself. At that point, all of us lose. You'd have a program that doesn't reflect how Alwyn and his team train their clients at Results Fitness, or how Alwyn and I train ourselves (and have for decades), or how we think most of you will achieve the best possible results.

While I'm on the topic, I understand that some of the most popular fitness programs and trainers promise amazing results with body-weight-only workouts or with just one type of equipment—bands, dumbbells, barbell, kettlebells, stripper pole . . .

255

Alwyn has a very simple way of answering the What about this? or Why not that? questions: "We're talking about objects," he says. "An object is not a system."

I once asked Stuart Phillips, a professor of exercise science at McMaster University in Hamilton, Ontario, if there's really any difference between exercise tools. "Your muscles don't know whether you're lifting free weights, machine weights, or your own body weight," he told me in an email. "Strength can come from any routine [or type of] equipment, especially when a decent effort is involved." (Phillips's thoughts about the role of effort in strength-training success are included in Chapter 2.)

Yes, you can build a system around an object, and many do for the obvious commercial reasons. But is that the best way to train when you have no financial stake in any particular product? Absolutely not. "If you only do one thing, you'll get better at that one thing," Phillips said. "But for me, it gets boring."

And here's an inside secret: The people who use their own physiques as proof that their object-based system is superior almost certainly *did not build their physiques with that system.* This fundamental deception goes all the way back to Charles Atlas. Atlas, whose original name was Angelo Siciliano, was an early 20th-century bodybuilder who sold millions of young men on the magic of "dynamic tension," a mail-order program of body-weight exercises and lifestyle tips. He was by all reports a genuinely nice man, but he was a well-known lifter before he began marketing his program, and some of his contemporaries objected to his claim that he owed his physique to dynamic tension.

With that out of the way, let's talk about the equipment you need, and a few things you may want.

How to Shop for Home Gym Equipment

Iron is iron. There's no reason secondhand equipment won't work as well as new stuff. A few specific tips:

- Start by looking at the price of new gear in stores or online. We highly recommend performbetter.com for just about anything you need.
- Once you have the full retail price, look around for discounts, as well as resale sites like eBay.
- No matter where you buy, always factor in shipping costs. Weights, by definition, weigh a lot. That makes them expensive to ship. It might be cheaper to pay full price with free shipping, if it's offered.

- The best bargains you'll find, if you're lucky enough to stumble into them, are at garage sales or on Craigslist. Shipping won't be an issue, as long as you have a car or truck to haul it away.

Dumbbells

You have three options:

Selectorized dumbbells give you a pair of handles that are usually 5 or 10 pounds each. Those handles fit into a mechanism that allows you to select weights up to the limit of the set. My gym has heavy-duty sets of PowerBlocks (the original and probably still the best example) that go up to 90 pounds each. At the company's website (powerblock.com) you'll see products that go even higher.

Advantages: You get a complete, versatile set of dumbbells that takes up just a few square feet of space. They have comfortable grips and are easy to use.

Disadvantages: A 50-pound set is at least $300 new, and if you want the stand (which is both useful and really nice-looking), that's another $150 at full retail.

Fixed-weight dumbbells can be much cheaper, especially if you buy them used. Just be sure you get them in pairs, and that you include weights that are heavier than what you can currently use in your workouts. You *will* get stronger than you are now, and you need to plan for that.

Advantages: You can buy what you need, when you need them.

Disadvantages: From the beginning you'll need a range of dumbbells—light for shoulder presses, somewhat heavier for rows, and heavier still for goblet squats. Each increase in strength means you'll need heavier weights to accommodate it and get even stronger. That creates potential organization, budget, and storage issues.

Adjustable dumbbell handles and weight plates are by far the worst option. I've used them at home, by necessity, and they're a complete pain in the ass. Either the collars are too loose, and the weights slide around, or they're so tight it's a struggle to change the weights between sets and exercises.

Barbell and Weight Plates

There are two types:

A *standard barbell* is an inch thick, 5 to 7 feet long, and usually weighs 10 pounds. If you buy a 110-pound set, you get the bar plus 90 pounds of weight plates, plus the aforementioned dumbbell handles, along with some collars to secure the plates on the bar. That's how I started, when I was thirteen, and I'm sure there are tens of millions of men and women who did the same.

Advantages: It's cheap ($100 or less for a beginner set) and easy to grip the bar if you have small hands.

Disadvantages: It's not great for deadlifts (the bar sits low to the ground), and if you share the equipment with any males in your household, they may quickly outgrow it.

An *Olympic barbell* is 2 inches wide at the ends, where the weights slide on. The bar is usually 7 feet long and weighs 45 pounds. You'll often find 300-pound sets that sell for around $300. Of course that's a lot more than you need right away, but might be useful down the road. (We've heard from readers who can now deadlift even more than that.)

Advantages: Once you can deadlift 135 pounds (the bar plus a 45-pound plate on each side), the bar will be 8.75 inches above the floor, which is the standard for a deadlift. Another benefit: The plates themselves can be used for resistance on some exercises. For example, you can do a goblet squat holding a weight plate against your chest.

Disadvantages: This is a very big set of equipment. You need to clear out some space to lift a seven-foot barbell, and you need a plan for storing the weights. You can get a five- or six-foot Olympic barbell, which will weigh 25 to 30 pounds and work just as well. But you'll have to buy the bar separately from plates—in other words, no discount for buying it as part of a set. Expect to pay at least $100.

Squat Rack with Chin-Up Bar

Not many beginners can do sets of chin-ups. For most women, it takes a while to build up to the first one. But you'll still find ways to use the horizontal bar at the top of the squat rack. It's a perfect attachment point for bands and a suspension system. The vertical support beams also provide anchor points for bands. You don't need a suspension system (which I'll discuss in a moment) to start, but bands (which I'll also get to shortly) will come in handy for several exercises.

It's called a squat rack because it has supports for a barbell, which allows you to do front and back squats. You won't do those exercises at the beginning of Alwyn's program, but you will do inverted rows—an exercise that looks like the mirror image of a push-up—and for that you'll need to rest a barbell on the supports.

Speaking of which, you can also use the setup I just described for elevated push-ups, which many of you will need to do before you can manage traditional push-ups on the floor.

A decent rack will be about 4 feet wide, 3 feet deep, and perhaps 7 feet tall.

A new one will cost several hundred dollars. I know that's a large chunk of money, which is why I think most new lifters will do best with at least a trial membership at a health club. That said, a lot of readers have found ways to train at home without a rack, especially in the first few months of the program. It's not perfect, but what is?

Bench, Box, Steps

It's good to have a traditional weight-lifting bench, one that's padded and 18 inches high. Along with the obvious bench presses, you can rest a hand on the bench for one-arm rows, or elevate your hands or feet on the bench for push-up and plank variations. You can also use it for step-ups, especially if you're tall or just have long legs.

Steps and boxes of other heights will come in handy. You don't need specialized equipment, as long as it's solid. You can use a staircase in your home for step-ups. You also might be able to find some adjustable aerobics steps at a garage sale; those work well for a variety of exercises.

Cable, Bands, Tubing

Cable exercises like rows and pulldowns are among the hardest to replicate at home. You can do the same movements with resistance bands and tubing, and they certainly work. The challenge is acquiring a range of bands to provide greater resistance as you get stronger.

I highly recommend getting some mini bands, which are used in Walk with Mini Band, shown in Chapter 11. They're typically 9 inches long and 2 inches wide, and come in four different tensions, which are color coded. Yellow has the lightest tension, followed by green, blue, and black. You'll find lots of options at perform better.com. I bought mine there on sale. (Don't tell my wife, but I think I paid more for shipping than I did for the bands.) You should be able to get an entire set for less than $15.

Mats and Padding

If you work out on a concrete floor in your garage or basement, you'll want some kind of padding to protect your elbows and knees on planks and kneeling exercises.

Clock or Timer

Some of Alwyn's core exercises, shown in Chapter 12, and all of his interval drills, described in Chapters 7 and 8, require you to time your sets. My all-time favorite interval timer was the $20 Gymboss (gymboss.com). When mine broke, I tried some free iPhone apps, but none worked as well as the Gymboss (including the company's own app). Now I simply use the stopwatch that came with my phone.

Suspension System

You'll see a lot of suspended exercises throughout *Strong*. Alwyn uses them in most of his workouts with most of his clients. You can attach a suspension trainer to a chin-up bar (as we do in the photos), a ceiling beam in your basement, a tree branch, or a swing set. You don't need one to begin the program—we show alternatives for most exercises—but you'll want one eventually. We use a TRX in the photos, which is the best known but also pricey, at $190 for a package that includes a DVD. You can buy cheaper alternatives (some *much* cheaper), and they may work equally well. You should also be able to find used equipment on eBay. The TRX is so well made that a secondhand device should be just as good as new.

Swiss Ball

Alwyn doesn't use the Swiss ball (aka stability, physio, or exercise ball) much anymore at Results Fitness. When the goal is to create some instability, he and his trainers prefer the TRX. But I still use one from time to time in my own workouts, for basically the same reasons we use it in *Strong* (not to mention all five NROL books). It's an easy, inexpensive way to add options for home workouts. You can find one online or at any sporting-goods store, usually for $20 or less.

Foam Roller

A foam roller is a cheap, convenient tool to help you work out the kinks that accumulate in your muscles. A basic one—18 inches long, 6 inches thick—will cost about $15. Today you can find more expensive options. Maybe they work better, but I wouldn't know. I still use the original.

Kettlebells

Finding kettlebells is no longer the challenge it was just a few years ago. They're everywhere, in all sizes and colors. The challenge is to get enough of them to accommodate your increasing strength. If you're an absolute beginner, you can start with a 15-pounder for swings, which you'll quickly outgrow. It's not useless at that point; it'll come in handy later for shoulder presses. But to keep doing swings, you'll need to move up. For exercises like the single-arm deadlift (shown in Chapter 13), you'll need one that's quite a bit heavier. Same with carries.

Another challenge is buying them in pairs. Even in commercial gyms it's rare to find pairs of kettlebells for exercises like the front squat in Chapter 13, or the carries shown in Chapter 15.

Sliding Discs

Valslides, which cost $30 and are shown in several exercises in Chapter 12, have plastic on the bottom and a rubber grip on top. They're great on carpet. For wood and tile floors, you'll need booties to reduce friction. They cost $5. Other companies now make similar products that sell for less. If you train in a gym, you can use a slide board. We understand that lots of readers prefer even cheaper options, like furniture sliders for carpeted floors. (You can find them at Home Depot or Lowe's.) Others use towels on wood or tile. Alwyn doesn't doubt that they work for some people in some situations, but he cautions that all exercise carries some risk. The risk rises when you do weight-bearing exercises without equipment designed for that purpose.

Ab Wheel

An ab wheel is basically a lawnmower wheel with handles on the sides, which you can buy online or in a sporting-goods store for $10 or less. Don't rush out to get one; you won't need it until Stage 8, the second-to-last program in *Strong*. The photo in Chapter 12 shows a more elaborate (and expensive) version of the wheel, one with foot straps for doing a long list of core exercises, including some we show in *Strong* that use Valslides or a TRX.

Heart-Rate Monitor

In the more advanced workouts, Alwyn recommends using a heart-rate monitor to determine when to stop one interval and begin the next. As explained in detail in Chapter 7, you don't have to use one. If you decide you want one, Alwyn recommends a basic chest-strap model from Polar, the Finnish company that patented the first wireless heart-rate monitor and has led the category as long as the category has existed. The H1, which you can find online for about $40, gives you heart-rate-zone alerts as described on page 66.

Medicine Balls, Weighted Vests, Etc.

Other items, like medicine balls and weighted vests, are luxury items when you begin a program (especially a vest that costs at least $100). But over time they come in handy and are fun to play around with.

Appendix C
How Much Weight Should I Use?

EXPERIENCED LIFTERS KNOW THERE'S NEVER A good answer to this question. You need to choose different weights for each exercise, and the weights you choose need to challenge you within the parameters of that day's workout. That's going to be different for everybody. Two novice lifters starting this program might be the same gender, size, and age, and yet they might use different loads for every exercise. One might be stronger than her hypothetical friend in her upper body but weaker in the lower body. One might have better stability and balance. And once we get to a certain age, all of us have aches, pains, and other limitations.

Take this from me: When you begin a new program, no matter how long you've been training, you'll almost never pick the perfect weight for each exercise, in each rep range.

But what's the perfect weight?

In the Stage 1 workouts, Alwyn has you do 2 sets of 12 reps of each exercise. The perfect weight will feel pretty heavy by the time you get to the 12th rep. On the first set, it should feel as if you could do *maybe* one or two more, but no more than two.

On the second set, the final rep should feel like the last one you can do without compromising your form (which you never want to do as a beginner).

The odds of choosing that perfect weight for any exercise, much less all of them, are about zero. Instead you have to work your way through a process of trial and error, one you'll have plenty of chances to practice in the *Strong* program.

Let's say you're doing the dumbbell goblet squat in Stage 1. You start with a 20-pound dumbbell. Even though it's an unfamiliar exercise, you can tell after just a few reps that 20 pounds is too light. Now what?

We'll call that first set a warm-up. Do 8 to 10 reps, return the weight, and choose a heavier one. But you're torn between the 25- and the 30-pounder. When in doubt, stay conservative. Choose the 25-pounder, and do your first set of 12 reps.

Still feel easy? No problem. Do the next exercise in the workout (dumbbell row), rest, and use 30 pounds for the second and final set of goblet squats. This time it feels more like a real exercise, but you still get all 12 reps. Again, no problem. Mark it in your log and move on.

The next time you do Workout A in Stage 1, you'll start with 35 pounds for goblet squats. If you easily get 12 reps, use 40 pounds for the second set.

But let's say 35 feels heavier than you expected, and you barely get 12 reps. Stick with 35 for the second set, even if it means you do only 9 or 10 reps. Use the same weight the next time you do Workout A, with the goal of getting 12 in both sets. And then you repeat the process.

At first it'll seem intimidating to go through this trial and error for every exercise in the program. But it's not. You'll quickly get good at guessing a likely weight to start out with. If you choose wrong, you'll know by the second or third rep, and learn to adjust on the fly.

There's even a hidden benefit to the process: You pick up, carry, and replace more weights in each workout, which adds to the total amount of work you do. The more times you guess wrong, the more calories you burn.

Two important guidelines:

- For any exercise, it's *always* better to start light and move up quickly, rather than start with too much weight and risk hurting yourself before you're comfortable with the movement pattern.
- That said, you must approach every set of every exercise with the goal of getting stronger. That's the only way the program works. Never settle for a lighter weight if you think you could do the same sets and reps with a heavier one.

Notes

Introduction: You Aren't Who You Used to Be

No reason to give women different advice: National Strength and Conditioning Association, "Strength Training for Female Athletes: A Position Paper: Part I," *NSCA Journal* 1989; 11(4): 43–55. National Strength and Conditioning Association, "Strength Training for Female Athletes: A Position Paper: Part II," *NSCA Journal* 1989; 11(5): 29–36. Jan Todd, "The Origins of Strength Training for Female Athletes in North America," *Iron Game History* 1992; 2(2): 4–14.

Facebook group: Dana's group is called The New Rules of Lifting for Women, Abs, Life & Supercharged. You can join by going to the page and requesting access. (That hurdle is made necessary by the spammers and assorted nut jobs who inevitably show up wherever people congregate online.) The original Facebook group is The New Rules of Lifting for Women: Lift Like a Man, Look Like a Goddess, run by Lisa Lilge (who's quoted in Chapter 15).

Success of NROL for Women: I wrote about this in a blog post: "The Book That Lived" (louschuler.com, April 22, 2014).

Chapter 1. Why Strength Matters

Importance of muscularity to men: Believe it or not, I read three studies for that simple observation: Lassek and Gaulin, "Costs and Benefits of Fat-Free Muscle Mass in Men: Relationship to Mating Success, Dietary Requirements, and Native Immunity," *Evolution and Human Behavior* 2009; 30: 322–328. Sell et al., "Formidability and the Logic of Human Anger," *Proceedings of the National Academy of Sciences USA* 2009; 106(35): 15073–15078. Sell et al., "The Importance of Physical Strength to Human Males," *Human Nature* 2012; 23: 30–44.

Benefits of strength: All the results mentioned were summarized in these studies: Artero et al., "Effects of Muscular Strength on Cardiovascular Risk Factors and Prognosis," *Journal of Cardiopulmonary Rehabilitation and Prevention* 2012; 32(6): 351–358. Phillips and Winett, "Uncomplicated Resistance Training and Health-Related Outcomes: Evidence for a Public Health Mandate," *Current Sports Medicine Reports* 2010; 9(4): 208–213. Mason et al., "Musculoskeletal Fitness and Weight Gain in Canada," *Medicine & Science in Sports & Exercise* 2007; 39(1): 38–43.

I tried running several times: For more about my sad history as a failed jogger and some useful information about how to do better than I did, please check out "Is Your Body Made for Running?" (menshealth.com, July 12, 2014).

Squat strength: For the comments on squat strength, I started with *Essentials of Strength Training and Conditioning*, 2nd ed. (Human Kinetics, 2000), p. 309. It's the official textbook of the National Strength and Conditioning Association, through which Alwyn and I are both certified. I also used "Insight for Strength Coaches: Power, Full Squats, Correlations, and Training Studies," by Bret Contreras (bretcontreras.com, September 27, 2013).

Ivy Russell's deadlift: Jan Todd, 1992.

Chapter 2. Why Muscle Matters

Muscle as an organ system: Demontis et al., "The Influence of Skeletal Muscle on Systemic Aging and Lifespan," *Aging Cell* 2013; 12: 943–949. Avin et al., "Skeletal Muscle As a Regulator of the Longevity Protein, Klotho," *Frontiers in Physiology* 2014; 5: article 189.

Any method of resistance training: Phillips and Winett, 2010.

Rate of muscle growth: Seynnes et al., "Early Skeletal Muscle Hypertrophy and Architectural Changes in Response to High-Intensity Resistance Training," *Journal of Applied Physiology* 2007; 102: 368–373. It was by necessity a small study, with just seven subjects. But two of them were women, which is important because groundbreaking muscle hypertrophy studies typically use male subjects.

Physical activity and longevity: Reimers et al., "Does Physical Activity Increase Life Expectancy? A Review of the Literature," *Journal of Aging Research* 2012; 2012: Article ID 243958. Samitz et al., "Domains of Physical Activity and All-Cause Mortality: Systematic Review and Dose-Response Meta-Analysis of Cohort Studies," *International Journal of Epidemiology* 2011; 40: 1382–1400.

MET values of exercise: Ainsworth et al., "Compendium of Physical Activities: An Update of Activity Codes and MET Intensities," *Medicine & Science in Sports & Exercise* 2000; 32 (9 Supplemental): S498–S504. (There's a 2011 update, which I don't have. I've used the 2000 version in countless articles and books, so switching to the later version feels like abandoning an old friend.)

Ratio of muscle to bone: *Sports Gene*, by David Epstein (Current, 2013), p. 124.

Bone growth: Chad Waterbury, "Bare Bones Physiology" (chadwaterbury.com, September 8, 2014).

Male and female comparisons: Lassek and Gaulin, 2009. National Strength and Conditioning Association, part I 1989.

Muscle hypertrophy: Stuart Phillips, "A Brief Review of Critical Processes in Exercise-Induced Muscular Hypertrophy," *Sports Medicine* 2014; 44 (Supplement 1): S71–S77. Phillips et al., "Mixed Muscle Protein Synthesis and Breakdown After Resistance Exercise in Humans," *American Journal of Physiology* 1997; 272 (1, Part 1): E99–E107. Brad Schoenfeld, "The Mechanisms of Muscle Hypertrophy and Their Application to Resistance Exercise," *Journal of Strength and Conditioning Research* 2010; 24(10): 2857–2872.

Chapter 3. Why Weight Control (*Not* Weight Loss) Matters

Fraudulent advice about weight loss: Ann La Berge, "How the Ideology of Low Fat Conquered America," *Journal of the History of Medicine* 2008; 63(2): 139–177.

Average weight for adult women in United States: The original chart appeared in *The New Rules of Lifting for Life* (Avery, 2012), p. 228. I got the idea from "Poor Choices, Not Aging, Pack on Pounds," by Nancy Helmich, *USA Today*, June 23, 2011. The most recent numbers were from "Anthropometric Reference Data for Children and Adults: United States, 2007–2010." *Vital and Health Statistics*, Series 11, Number 252.

Losing strength and muscle mass: *All About Muscle*, by Irwin Siegel (Demos, 2000), p. 58.

Calories burned at rest: Hoffmans et al., "Resting Metabolic Rate in Obese and Normal-Weight Women," *International Journal of Obesity* 1979; 3(2): 111–118.

Metabolism: Most of this is basic textbook information that I've used in previous NROL books.

Average calories: Ford and Dietz, "Trends in Energy Intake Among Adults in the United States: Findings from NHANES," *American Journal of Clinical Nutrition* 2013; 97: 848–853. It's important to note that these calculations are based on self-reported food intake, which means the actual averages are probably at least 10 percent higher.

Net weight gain: Rosenbaum and Leibel, "Adaptive Thermogenesis in Humans," *International Journal of Obesity* 2010; 34: S47–S55. Cook et al., "Relation Between Holiday Weight Gain and Total Energy Expenditure Among 40- to 69-Year-Old Men and Women (OPEN Study)," *American Journal of Clinical Nutrition* 2012: 95: 726–731. I admit this is a self-share: I used this data to make the exact same point in the introduction to *Lean Muscle Diet* (Rodale, 2014, p. x), which I wrote with Alan Aragon. I also used it in a magazine feature: "Santa Claus: The Makeover," *Men's Health*, December 2013, pp. 140–147.

Adaptive thermogenesis: Leibel et al., "Changes in Energy Expenditure Resulting from Altered Body Weight," *New England Journal of Medicine* 1995; 332: 621–628. Camps et al., "Weight Loss, Weight Maintenance, and Adaptive Thermogenesis," *American Journal of Clinical Nutrition* 2013: 97: 990–994.

Weight regain: Rosenbaum and Leibel, 2010.

Typical sentence in weight-loss article: The sentence I used is from "Which Diet Will Help You Lose the Most Weight?" by Emily Oster (fivethirtyeight.com, October 14, 2014).

History of weight standards: Kuczmarski and Flegal, "Criteria for Definition of Overweight in Transition: Background and Recommendation for the United States," *American Journal of Clinical Nutrition* 2000: 72(5): 1074–1081.

Katherine Flegal: At the beginning of *The End of Overeating* (Rodale, 2009), author David Kessler, M.D., describes how Flegal came across the data in the National Health and Nutrition Examination Survey (NHANES), which was conducted from 1988 to 1991. She published the data in the *American Journal of Clinical Nutrition* in 1994. Six years later, in 2000, she published the study cited in the previous note ("History of Weight Standards") to explain the new criteria for overweight and obesity. Thirteen years after *that*, she published the report cited in the following note.

Body weight and mortality: Flegal and Kalantar-Zadeh, "Perspective: Overweight, Mortality, and Survival," *Obesity* 2013; 21(9): 1744–1745.

Exercise is underrated: The article I wrote for *Men's Health* was called "Smash Fat Faster" (November 2013, pp. 146–149; menshealth.com, November 25, 2013). It was based on this study: Bernard Gutin, "How Can We Help People to Develop Lean and Healthy Bodies? A New Perspective," *Research Quarterly for Exercise and Sport* 2013; 84: 1–5. I came across the study in the June 2013 issue of *Strength & Conditioning Research*, a monthly roundup put together by Bret Contreras and Chris Beardsley (strengthandconditioningresearch.com). It costs $10 a month and has become indispensable to me as a journalist who struggles to keep up with all the areas I write about.

Women who train more also eat more: Lee et al., "Physical Activity and Weight Gain Prevention," *Journal of the American Medical Association* 2010; 303(12): 1173–1179.

Metabolic rate and appetite: Caudwell et al., "Resting Metabolic Rate Is Associated with Hunger, Self-Determined Meal Size, and Daily Energy Intake and May Represent a Marker for Appetite," *American Journal of Clinical Nutrition* 2013: 97: 7–14.

Chapter 4. Why Protein Is the Key to a Successful Diet

Protein: Hubert Vickery, "The Origin of the Word 'Protein,'" *Yale Journal of Biology and Medicine* 1950; 22(5): 387–393.

Protein in weight-loss research: Morrison et al., "Homeostatic Regulation of Protein Intake: In Search of a Mechanism," *American Journal of Physiology. Regulatory, Integrative, and Comparative Physiology* 2012; 302(8): R917–R928.

Quality of protein in fast food: Prayson et al., "Fast Food Hamburgers: What Are We Really Eating?" *Annals of Diagnostic Pathology* 2008; 12(6): 406–409. "Taco Bell's Seasoned Meat Is Only 88 Percent Beef. It Should Be Way, Way Less," by L. V. Anderson (slate.com, May 1, 2014).

Protein leverage hypothesis: *The Nature of Nutrition: A Unifying Framework from Animal Adaptation to Human Obesity*, by Stephen Simpson and David Raubenheimer (Princeton University Press, 2012). Simpson and Raubenheimer were coauthors of this study: Gosby et al., "Protein Leverage and Energy Intake," *Obesity Reviews* 2014; 15: 183–191. The 30 percent threshold for leverage to occur was found here: Martens et al., "Protein Leverage Affects Energy Intake of High-Protein Diets in Humans," *American Journal of Clinical Nutrition* 2013: 97: 86–93.

Diet comparisons: Wycherley et al., "Effects of Energy-Restricted High-Protein, Low-Fat Compared with Standard-Protein, Low-Fat Diets: A Meta-Analysis of Randomized Controlled Trials," *American Journal of Clinical Nutrition* 2012: 96: 1281–1298.

Target body weight: This is the system used by Alan Aragon, my coauthor on *Lean Muscle Diet*, where you can find the actual formula Alan uses with clients. Although the book was written for men, the basic information applies to both genders. If you've read the book, you can find specific tips for women in "Frequently Asked Questions About *The Lean Muscle Diet*" (alanaragon.com, January 6, 2015).

Personal preference: Johnston et al., "Comparison of Weight Loss Among Named Diet

Programs in Overweight and Obese Adults: A Meta-Analysis." *Journal of the American Medical Association* 2014; 312(9): 923–933.

Protein timing: Arciero et al., "Increased Protein Intake and Meal Frequency Reduces Abdominal Fat During Energy Balance and Energy Deficit," *Obesity* 2013; 21: 1357–1366. Arciero et al., "Timed Daily Ingestion of Whey Protein and Exercise Training Reduces Visceral Adipose Tissue Mass and Improves Insulin Resistance: The PRISE Study," *Journal of Applied Physiology* 2014; 117(1): 1–10.

Maximum effective dose of protein: I covered all this in greater detail in Chapter 5 of *The New Rules of Lifting Supercharged* (Avery, 2012), pp. 42–50.

Post-workout protein recommendations: Stuart Phillips, 2014.

Exercise and appetite: Martins et al., "Effects of Exercise on Gut Peptides, Energy Intake, and Appetite," *Journal of Endocrinology* 2007; 193(2): 251–258. King et al., "Exercise-Induced Suppression of Appetite: Effects on Food Intake and Implications for Energy Balance," *European Journal of Clinical Nutrition* 1994; 48(10): 715–724. Schubert et al., "Acute Exercise and Hormones Related to Appetite Regulation: A Meta-Analysis," *Sports Medicine* 2014; 44(3): 387–403.

Leucine: *NROL Supercharged*, pp. 47–48.

Benefits of whey supplements: Sousa et al., "Dietary Whey Protein Lessens Several Risk Factors for Metabolic Diseases: A Review," *Lipids in Health and Disease* 2012; 11: 67. Bendtsen et al., "Effect of Dairy Proteins on Appetite, Energy Expenditure, Body Weight, and Composition: A Review of the Evidence from Controlled Clinical Trials," *Advances in Nutrition* 2013; 4: 418–438.

Soy protein compares favorably to whey: *Dietary Protein and Resistance Exercise*, edited by Lonnie Lowery and Jose Antonio (CRC Press, 2012), pp. 109–110.

Chapter 5. Why All This Still Seems So Confusing

Post-workout muscle breakdown and synthesis: *Dietary Protein and Resistance Exercise*, pp. 31, 87.

Myth of spot reduction: "Spot Reduction: One Final Attempt to Kill the Myth," by Tom Kelso (breakingmuscle.com, September 29, 2013). "For the Millionth Time, Spot Reduction Is a Myth!" by Bret Contreras (bretcontreras.com, August 14, 2013). Both articles reference this study: Ramirez-Campillo et al., "Regional Fat Changes Induced by Localized Muscle Endurance Resistance Training," *Journal of Strength and Conditioning Research* 2013; 27(8): 2219–2224. Bret's article also makes an important point: While it's impossible to burn fat from specific spots with targeted exercises, the opposite is true for building muscle. Strength training is very much site specific, meaning you don't build your arms with squats and you don't build your legs with bench presses. But with a strenuous workout that changes your body composition, squats could indeed help you lose fat in your arms, along with your legs and every other place where it's stored.

Old science facts: "Cuckoo for Cocoa Puffs: Why Are We So Sure That Breakfast Is the Most Important Meal of the Day?" by Daniel Engber (slate.com, September 9, 2013). "Three Squares a Day vs. a Day of Smaller Meals: Which Is Better for Healthy Weight Loss?" by Jill Adams (washingtonpost.com, August 26, 2013). "The Myth of Ripped Muscles and Calorie Burns," by James Fell (latimes.com, May 16, 2011). "A Pound of Muscle Burns 30–50 Kcal/ Day, Really . . ." National Council on Strength & Fitness (ncsf.org). "You Don't Need Eight Glasses of Water a Day," by Emily Oster (fivethirtyeight.com, September 30, 2014).

Weight-loss math: Kevin Hall, "What Is the Required Energy Deficit per Unit Weight Loss?" *International Journal of Obesity* 2008; 32(3): 573–576. Hall et al., "Quantification of the Effect of Energy Imbalance on Body Weight," *The Lancet* 2011; 378: 826–837. Thomas et al., "Can a Weight Loss of One Pound a Week Be Achieved with a 3,500 Kcal Deficit? Commentary on a Commonly Accepted Rule," *International Journal of Obesity* 2013; 37(12): 1611–1613. Hall and Chow, "Why Is the 3,500 Kcal per Pound Weight Loss Rule Wrong?" *International Journal of Obesity* 2013; 37(12): 1614.

Moderation and longevity: I could dig up specific sources, but really this comes from seeing the same basic data points in lots of studies over the years. The people who live the longest life in the United States tend to be well educated and affluent, and as such they follow trends when there appears to be a clear health benefit. They were the first to quit smoking (and discourage their children from starting), to wear seat belts, and to use sunscreen. (Yes, I'm old enough to remember when these were all new ideas.) Same with nutrition: When told to avoid saturated fat, they did. When told nuts and yogurt and exotic fruits and vegetables were healthy, they started eating them.

When groups become cults: As we were doing final edits for *Strong,* I wrote an article about vaccines ("Vaccines Are Not Controversial. They're Safe. They Work. That's It," menshealth .com, February 5, 2015). The article led me to *The Panic Virus,* by Seth Mnookin (Simon & Schuster, 2011). Even if you don't care about vaccines, the book is worth reading just for the insights you'll find in Chapter 16, titled "Cognitive Biases and Availability Cascades." Mnookin offers the best explanation I've seen for why people cling so fiercely to concepts long after they've debunked. One small sample: "The anonymity and lack of friction inherent in the online world also mean that a small number of committed activists—or even an especially zealous individual—can create the impression that a fringe viewpoint has broad support." Best of all, Mnookin details the published research that supports some of the points I attempt to make in this chapter.

Chapter 6. How the System Works

Goblet squat: For more background, I recommend reading "Goblet Squats 101," by Dan John (t-nation.com, March 3, 2011).

Chapter 8. Phase Two: Demand

Mark Wahlberg is jealous: Search Google Images for "Mark Wahlberg home gym" if you don't get the reference.

Resistance training + intervals for body composition: In *The New Rules of Lifting for Women* (Avery, 2007), pp. 21–23, we mentioned the afterburn effect of a strength workout and looked at the potential for increasing resting metabolic rate. In *The New Rules of Lifting* (Avery, 2006), pp. 254–257, I wrote about energy flux, which is the idea that exercising more and eating more has a bigger effect on your metabolism than either in isolation. I hadn't thought about the latter idea in years, but I was reminded of it when I read about the following doctoral dissertation by a graduate student at Colorado State University: Rebecca Foright, "A High Energy Flux State Attenuates the Weight Loss–Induced Energy Gap by Acutely Decreasing Hunger and Increasing Satiety and Resting Metabolic Rate." I found the abstract at gradworks.umi.com, but by the time you read this there might be a published study based on the research.

Perfect vs. good: Which man said it is open to debate. It's generally attributed to Voltaire, but Professor Wikipedia notes that Confucius, Aristotle, and Shakespeare all expressed a similar idea. Common sense tells us lots of women have had the same thought, and one or two may have written it down somewhere.

Chapter 9. Phase Three: Display

RPE for strength training: I learned about the system from Bret Contreras in a blog post titled "Three Tips for Faster Strength Gains" (bretcontreras.com, November 17, 2014). The system originates with powerlifter and strength coach Mike Tuchscherer (reactivetraining systems.com).

Overhead press in Olympics: For a brief but authoritative look at the history, I recommend "The Manly Military Press," by Jim Schmitz (ironmind.com). Schmitz was coach of the U.S. Olympic weightlifting team in 1980, 1988, and 1992.

Dramatic metabolic response: The drop-set component of Alwyn's program is inspired, in part, by this study: Paoli et al., "High-Intensity Interval Resistance Training (HIRT) Influences Resting Energy Expenditure and Respiratory Ratio in Non-Dieting Individuals," *Journal of Translational Medicine* 2012; 10: 237. They used a different technique, which they call HIRT. Veteran lifters will recognize it as rest-pause training. It's similar to what Alwyn has you do, only without reducing the weight each set. In the study, a group of young male lifters were still burning calories about 25 percent faster a day after their HIRT workout. Specifically, they went from burning about 80 calories an hour before the workout to burning about 100 an hour 22 hours later. The workout itself took less than a half hour. You can find a detailed discussion of the study, including reasons to be slightly skeptical about the huge increase in metabolic rate, in "The Strange Tale of HIRT and the Afterburn Effect," by Christian Finn (muscleevo.net).

Chapter 10. Moves That Matter

"The results should be exactly the same": I mean this in reference to the general population of fitness enthusiasts. Advanced strength athletes in any discipline—bodybuilders, powerlifters, CrossFitters, Olympic weightlifters—will train in ways specific to their sport. That, in turn, will produce different visual results. The best example is bodybuilders vs. powerlifters. The former will focus on the mind–muscle connection, concentrating each contraction on the parts of muscles they want to develop. The latter will focus on techniques that allow them to lift the heaviest possible weights. CrossFitters and Olympic lifters also develop distinctive physiques based on the demands of their sport.

You could extend this to athletes like gymnasts, tennis players, and mixed martial artists, where strength training contributes to a type of physique we associate with those sports. That said, I don't mean to imply that you can look like an athlete by training like that athlete. Serena Williams and Maria Sharapova didn't achieve their unique frames because they play and train for tennis. I'm just saying there's a level of muscularity and type of conditioning we associate with different sports. Rock climbers don't look like bodybuilders, and you rarely see a bodybuilder climbing rocks.

Nick Tumminello: The quote—"Don't fit yourself to exercises, fit exercises to you"—can be found in several of his articles, including this one: "Personal Training: Four Principles of Exercise Selection" (nicktumminello.com, November 12, 2014). Nick is also the author of *Strength Training for Fat Loss* (Human Kinetics, 2014).

Chapter 11. RAMP

Self-myofascial release: "Foam Rolling Edition," by Chris Beardsley, in *Strength & Conditioning Research* (December 2014). Chris's analysis was based on several studies, including this one: Mohr et al., "Effect of Foam Rolling and Static Stretching on Passive Hip-Flexion Range of Motion," *Journal of Sport Rehabilitation* 2014; 23(4): 296–299.

Breathing: For an authoritative and highly detailed argument for why it's important to fix your breathing, I recommend "Diaphragmatic Breathing Through Pulling vs. Through Pushing," by Dean Somerset (deansomerset.com, October 11, 2013).

Role of glutes in knee stability: I recommend two articles by Bret Contreras: "Glute Science" (bretcontreras.com, August 7, 2013) and "Exciting New Glute Research Pertaining to Knee Biomechanics in the Lunge" (bretcontreras.com, November 8, 2012). I realize the headlines aren't especially enticing, but Bret's love of all things related to glutes and biomechanics makes the articles more fun to read than you'd expect.

Chapter 12. Core Training

Core stability: The definition I use is a paraphrase of one stated in this study: Kibler et al., "The Role of Core Stability in Athletic Function," *Sports Medicine* 2006; 36(3): 189–198.

Back pain prevention: *Low Back Disorders*, by Stuart McGill (Human Kinetics, 2002), p. 143. The key quote: "Having strong abdominals does not necessarily provide the prophylactic effect that many hoped for. However, several works suggest that muscular endurance reduces the risk of future back troubles."

Back pain reduction: Stuber et al., "Core Stability Exercises for Low Back Pain in Athletes: A Systematic Review of the Literature," *Clinical Journal of Sport Medicine* 2014; 24(6): 448–456.

"That whole brevity thing": A nod to *The Big Lebowski*, possibly the greatest stoner comedy of all time, at least in the eyes of a nonstoner like me. Actual marijuana enthusiasts rank it ninth, according to "*High Times*' 40 Greatest Stoner Movies of All Time" (hightimes.com, May 29, 2014).

Muscle activation in rollouts and fallouts: Escamilla et al., "Core Muscle Activation During Swiss Ball and Traditional Abdominal Exercises," *Journal of Orthopaedic & Sports Physical Therapy* 2010; 40(5): 265–276. The study looked at a rollout with a Swiss ball, which, in terms of technique, is similar to three exercises Alwyn includes in *Strong*: Valslide pushaway, ab-wheel rollout, and suspended fallout. Activation of the rectus abdominis was higher than in any of the other nine exercises studied. Rollouts also worked the obliques (both internal and external) harder than sit-ups and crunches. I like this study because it used a mix of male and female college students to measure muscle activation and provide useful, widely applicable benchmarks.

Muscle activation in jackknife and pike: Escamilla et al., 2010. As with the rollout, muscle activation was measured on a Swiss ball.

Body saw, hanging leg and knee raise, walkout: McGill et al., "Muscle Activity and Spine Load During Anterior Chain Whole Body Linkage Exercises: The Body Saw, Hanging Leg Raise, and Walkout from a Pushup," *Journal of Sports Sciences* 2014; 11: 1–8. The technique used for the body saw is slightly different from ours; the researchers combined the movement we show with a knee tuck.

Muscle activation in push-up: Calatayud et al., "Muscle Activation During Pushups with Different Suspension Training Systems," *Journal of Sports Science and Medicine* 2014; 13: 502–510.

Chapter 13. Lower-Body Exercises

Front squats vs. back squats: Bird and Casey, "Exploring the Front Squat," *Strength and Conditioning Journal* 2012; 34(2): 27–33. See also *NROL Supercharged*, p. 14.

Box squat: For an explanation of why elite powerlifters do them: "Box Squatting Benefits," by Louie Simmons (westside-barbell.com, June 15, 2013). And for those most interested in muscle development: "Back Squats vs. Box Squats," by Dan Blewitt (t-nation.com, April 16, 2014).

Knee stress in box squat: Swinton et al., "A Biomechanical Comparison of the Traditional Squat, Powerlifting Squat, and Box Squat," *Journal of Strength and Conditioning Research* 2012; 26(7): 1805–1816. It's described here, in layman's terms: "Traditional Squat vs. Power-lifting Squat vs. Box Squat," by Bret Contreras (bretcontreras.com, April 14, 2012).

Strength vs. power: *NROL Supercharged*, pp. 28–29.

Muscles used in hex-bar deadlift: Swinton et al., "A Biomechanical Analysis of Straight and Hexagonal Bar Deadlifts Using Submaximal Loads," *Journal of Strength and Conditioning Research* 2011; 25(7): 2000–2009. See also *NROL Supercharged*, pp. 90 and 106.

Partial unilateral exercises: McCurdy et al., "The Effects of Short-Term Unilateral and Bilateral Lower-Body Resistance Training on Measures of Strength and Power," *Journal of Strength and Conditioning Research* 2005; 19(1): 9–15. Jones et al., "Effects of Unilateral and Bilateral Lower-Body Heavy Resistance Exercise on Muscle Activity and Testosterone Responses," *Journal of Strength and Conditioning Research* 2012; 26(4): 1094–1100.

Muscles used in step-up: Simenz et al., "Electromyographical Analysis of Lower-Extremity Muscle Activation During Variations of the Loaded Step-Up Exercise," *Journal of Strength and Conditioning Research* 2012; 26(12): 3398–3405.

Chapter 14. Upper-Body Exercises

Personal records in chest and shoulder presses: Because you asked, the records were 2 reps with 100 pounds in the dumbbell bench press, and 5 reps with 60 pounds in the dumbbell shoulder press. Before then, my records for those lifts were 2 reps with 95 and 5 with 55. In the barbell bench press, my record was a single rep with 260 pounds. A few days before setting my dumbbell records, I failed to lift 250.

Push-up facts: Suprak et al., "The Effect of Position on the Percentage of Body Mass Supported During Traditional and Modified Pushup Variants," *Journal of Strength and Conditioning Research* 2011; 25(2): 497–503. Ebben et al., "Kinetic Analysis of Several Variations of

Pushups," *Journal of Strength and Conditioning Research* 2011; 25(10): 2891–2894. Yet again, I learned about the first of these studies, and many others, from articles by Bret Contreras: "The Best Damn Pushups Article, Period!" by Bret and Elsbeth Vaino (t-nation.com, June 22, 2011), and "Pushup Research" (bretcontreras.com, June 23, 2011).

Muscle size: *All About Muscle*, p. xviii.

Suspended row: Fenwick et al., "Comparison of Different Rowing Exercises: Trunk Muscle Activation and Lumbar Spine Motion, Load, and Stiffness," *Journal of Strength and Conditioning Research* 2009; 23(2): 350–358.

Lat pulldown: Snyder and Leech, "Voluntary Increase in Latissimus Dorsi Muscle Activity During the Lat Pulldown Following Expert Instruction," *Journal of Strength and Conditioning Research* 2009; 23(8): 2204–2209. Lusk et al., "Grip Width and Forearm Orientation Effects on Muscle Activity During the Lat Pulldown," *Journal of Strength and Conditioning Research* 2010; 24(7): 1895–1900. Andersen et al., "Effects of Grip Width on Muscle Strength and Activation in the Lat Pulldown," *Journal of Strength and Conditioning Research* 2014; 28(4): 1135–1142.

Chapter 15. Intervals, Cardio, and the Perils of All of the Above

Strength training improves mobility: *Designing Resistance Training Programs*, 3rd ed, by Steven Fleck and William Kraemer (Human Kinetics, 2004), notes on pp. 145–146 that certain types of resistance training have been shown to increase flexibility.

Strength training improves cardiovascular fitness: James Timmons, "Variability in Training-Induced Skeletal Muscle Adaptation," *Journal of Applied Physiology* 2011; 11: 846–853. The specific statement: "[S]trength training can sometimes promote an improved VO$_2$max when endurance training does not."

Interval training benefits: Stephen Boutcher, "High-Intensity Intermittent Exercise and Fat Loss," *Journal of Obesity* 2011; article ID 868305.

Muscle development with sled push: Maddigan et al., "Lower Limb and Trunk Muscle Activation with Back Squats and Weighted Sled Apparatus," *Journal of Strength and Conditioning Research* 2014; 28(12): 3346–3353.

Benefits of loaded carries: McGill et al., "Comparison of Different Strongman Events: Trunk Muscle Activation and Lumbar Spine Motion, Load, and Stiffness," *Journal of Strength and Conditioning Research* 2009; 23(4): 1148–1161.

Dangers of sitting: "Killer Chairs," by James Levine (*Scientific American*, November 2014, pp. 34–35). Dr. Levine is the Mayo Clinic researcher who coined the acronym NEAT, for nonexercise activity thermogenesis, to explain how small movements, like fidgeting, contribute to weight management.

Fitness, health, and mortality: Paul Williams, "Physical Fitness and Activity As Separate Heart Disease Risk Factors: A Meta-Analysis," *Medicine & Science in Sports & Exercise* 2001; 33(5): 754–761.

Light activity and recovery: Mann et al., "High Responders and Low Responders: Factors Associated with Individual Variation in Response to Standardized Training," *Sports Medicine* 2014; 44(8): 1113–1124.

Alexander Juan Antonio Cortes: Alexander writes the "Lion in Iron" column at elitefts .com and is a coach at mountaindogdiet.com.

Interference effect: Wilson et al., "Concurrent Training: A Meta-Analysis Examining Interference of Aerobic and Resistance Exercises," *Journal of Strength and Conditioning Research* 2012; 26(8): 2293–2307.

Cycling and muscle growth: Lundberg et al., "Aerobic Exercise Does Not Compromise Muscle Hypertrophy Response to Short-Term Resistance Training," *Journal of Applied Physiology* 2013; 114: 81–89.

Greg Nuckols: Greg's website is strengtheory.com. I highly recommend his series on male–female differences in physiology and training effects, starting with "Gender Differences in Training and Metabolism" (strengtheory.com, January 11, 2015).

Eric Cressey: Eric describes what he learned about cardio for powerlifting in "My Top Five Powerlifting Mistakes" (ericcressey.com, July 15, 2014).

Appendix A: A Beginner's Guide to Lifting

Dave Draper: Dave was one of the top bodybuilders of the 1960s, winning Mr. Universe in 1966. He appeared on a couple of the shows I watched, including *The Monkees*, which is probably where I saw him. (Although I had a false memory of seeing him play a surfer on *Gilligan's Island*. That was a different guy.) I contacted him through his wife, Laree Draper. One of her companies, movementlectures.com, sells an audio presentation of mine called "The Hero's Journey into Fitness."

Appendix B: Strength-Training Equipment

Charles Atlas: I briefly mention Atlas in Chapter 3 of *The Lean Muscle Diet*, and get into the weeds of his backstory in the Notes on p. 280.

Index

Page numbers in **bold** indicate charts; numbers in *italic* indicate illustrations.

ALSO BY LOU SCHULER AND ALWYN COSGROVE

The series that has revolutionized weight lifting.

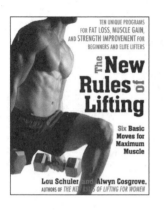

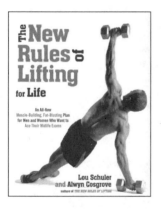

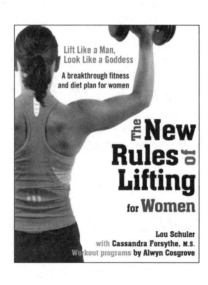

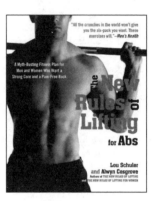

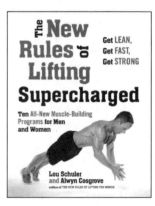

thenewrulesoflifting.com

AVERY